Teen Health Series

Diet Information For Teens, Fourth Edition

Diet Information For Teens,
Fourth Edition

Health Tips About Nutrition Fundamentals
And Eating Plans

Including Facts About Vitamins, Minerals, Food Additives,
And Weight-Related Concerns

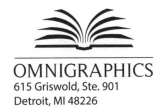

OMNIGRAPHICS
615 Griswold, Ste. 901
Detroit, MI 48226

Bibliographic Note
Because this page cannot legibly accommodate all the copyright notices, the Bibliographic Note portion of the Preface constitutes an extension of the copyright notice.

* * *

Omnigraphics
a part of Relevant Information
Keith Jones, *Managing Editor*

* * *

Copyright © 2017 Omnigraphics
ISBN 978-0-7808-1386-1
E-ISBN 978-0-7808-1410-3

Library of Congress Cataloging-in-Publication Data

Names: Omnigraphics, Inc.

Title: Diet information for teens: health tips about nutrition fundamentals and eating plans including facts about vitamins, minerals, food additives, and weight-related concerns.

Description: Fourth edition. | Detroit, MI: Omnigraphics, [2017] | Series: Teen health series | Includes bibliographical references and index.

Identifiers: LCCN 2016035858 (print) | LCCN 2016037213 (ebook) | ISBN 9780780813861 (hardcover: alk. paper) | ISBN 9780780814103 (ebook) | ISBN 9780780814103 (eBook)

Subjects: LCSH: Teenagers--Nutrition. | Teenagers--Health and hygiene. | Diet. | Health.

Classification: LCC RJ235 .D546 2017 (print) | LCC RJ235 (ebook) | DDC 613.20835--dc23

LC record available at https://lccn.loc.gov/2016035858

Table of Contents

Preface

Part One: Nutrition Fundamentals

Chapter 1——Dietary Guidelines 3

Chapter 2——Understanding Calories 7

Chapter 3——Understanding The Food Label 11

Chapter 4——Grains 23

Chapter 5——Vegetables 29

Chapter 6——Fruits 35

Chapter 7——The Dairy Group 41

Chapter 8——The Protein Group 47

Chapter 9——Oils..55

Chapter 10—Empty Calories 59

Chapter 11—Water: Meeting Your Daily Fluid Needs 63

Part Two: Vitamins And Minerals

Chapter 12—Vitamin A And Carotenoids 69

Chapter 13—B Vitamins 73

Chapter 14—Vitamin C 85

Chapter 15—Vitamin D...89

Chapter 16—Vitamin E 93

Chapter 17—Vitamin K 97

Chapter 18—Calcium 101

Chapter 19—Iron 107

Chapter 20—Magnesium... 111

Chapter 21—Zinc.. 115

Chapter 22—Other Important Minerals 119

Chapter 23—Multivitamin And Mineral (MVM) Dietary
Supplements.. 127

Chapter 24—What You Need To Know About Dietary
Supplements.. 131

Part Three: Other Elements Inside Food

Chapter 25—Sodium: Salt By Any Name 139

Chapter 26—Carbohydrates.. 147

Chapter 27—Sugars / Syrups (Added Sugars).................... 151

Chapter 28—Sugar Substitutes (High-Intensity Sweeteners) 153

Chapter 29—Which Fats Are Which? 157

Chapter 30—Food Ingredients, Additives, And Colors 161

Part Four: Smart Eating Plans

Chapter 31—MyPlate Nutrition Guide: Building a Healthy
Plate 171

Chapter 32—Eating Well To Live Well................................ 177

Chapter 33—Food Shopping Tips 187

Chapter 34—Eating Well While Eating Out 191

Chapter 35—Fast-Food Alternatives................................... 195

Chapter 36—Eating In The School Cafeteria..................... 201

Chapter 37—Healthy Snacking 205

Chapter 38—What You Should Know About Caffeine And
Energy Drinks.. 209

Chapter 39—Sports Supplements....................................... 215

Chapter 40—Healthy Eating For Vegans And Vegetarians 221

Part Five: Eating And Weight-Related Concerns

Chapter 41—Body Mass Index For Teens 229

Chapter 42—What's The Right Weight For My Height? 233

Chapter 43—Body Image And Self-Esteem 237

Chapter 44—Weight-Loss And Nutrition Myths............................. 241

Chapter 45—Choosing A Safe And Successful Weight-Loss
Program 247

Chapter 46—Should I Gain Weight? 253

Chapter 47—Health Fraud Awareness................................... 257

Chapter 48—Physical Activity And Health 261

Chapter 49—Reduce Screen Time 267

Part Six: Eating And Disease

Chapter 50—Disease Prevention Through Good Eating
Habits 273

Chapter 51—Heart Healthy Eating... 281

Chapter 52—The Childhood Obesity Problem 283

Chapter 53—Dealing With Celiac Disease 289

Chapter 54—Dealing With Diabetes...................................... 295

Chapter 55—Dealing With Food Allergies............................ 305

Chapter 56—Dealing With Lactose Intolerance 307

Chapter 57—Understanding Foodborne Illness 315

Chapter 58—Understanding Eating Disorders 325

Part Seven: If You Need More Information

Chapter 59—Cooking Tips And Resources............................ 335

Chapter 60—Eat Smart And Be Active As You Grow—Tips
For Teen Guys.. 339

Chapter 61—Eat Smart And Be Active As You Grow—Tips
For Teen Girls.. 341

Chapter 62—Resources For Dietary Information 343

Chapter 63—Resources For Fitness Information 349

Index 357

Preface

About This Book

The way adolescents spend their time can strongly influence their health later in life. Today's teens are exposed to an array of technological tools that they can use to connect with information. In fact, children and teens between the ages of 8 and 18 may spend up to 7 hours a day using media, such as watching television, playing video games, or using computers and cell phones. But, being so connected might be disconnecting them from the healthy diets their developing bodies need.

In the swirl of misleading and confusing nutrition information found in television advertisements and on the internet, it can be difficult for a teen to know what constitutes a proper diet. Rising rates of some health conditions, like diabetes and obesity, make it especially important that teens become educated about their dietary choices because what a teenager chooses to eat can have implications that last a lifetime.

Diet Information For Teens, Fourth Edition, provides updated information about healthy eating patterns and making smart dietary choices, including facts from the recently released *Dietary Guidelines for Americans* and the MyPlate food guidance system. The book discusses the essential components of a well-constructed diet and explains how major food groups— such as grains, vegetables, fruits, and protein foods—play an important role in providing the vitamins and minerals needed to maintain good health. Dietary elements that may need to be limited, such as caffeine, sugar, fat, and salt, are also discussed along with tips for reducing screen time, staying active, and addressing weight-related concerns. A special section on eating and disease provides information about foodborne illness, eating disorders, and disorders where dietary choices are an essential part of disease management procedures. The book concludes with cooking tips and directories of resources for dietary and fitness information.

How To Use This Book

This book is divided into parts and chapters. Parts focus on broad areas of interest; chapters are devoted to single topics within a part.

Part One: Nutrition Fundamentals looks at the most recently released *Dietary Guidelines for Americans* and explains dietary components. It discusses calorie requirements and energy balance, and it explains how nutrition facts labels can be used to help compare the nutrient contents of food items. Details about the individual food groups that comprise a healthy diet, including grains, vegetables, fruits, dairy and proteins, are also included.

Part Two: Vitamins And Minerals offers individual chapters focusing on the major vitamins—A, B, C, D, E, and K—and calcium, a mineral of special concern to growing teens. Each chapter discusses the role the nutrient plays in maintaining good health and gives examples of foods that are rich sources of the nutrient. Additional chapters provide facts about other important minerals and dietary supplements.

Part Three: Other Elements Inside Food discusses components of foods that are sometimes consumed in excess or that may be monitored carefully for specific purposes. These include salt, carbohydrates, sugars, and fats. Information about food additives and artificial sweeteners is also included.

Part Four: Smart Eating Plans talks about the MyPlate food guidance system and discusses ways to develop eating patterns that support a healthy lifestyle. It also offers suggestions for making healthy food choices in a variety of settings, including eating out, eating in the school cafeteria, and snacking. Facts about caffeine, energy drinks, and sports supplements are presented, and the part concludes with information for vegetarians and vegans.

Part Five: Eating And Weight-Related Concerns addresses readers who want to identify and maintain a healthy weight. It describes the body mass index (BMI), discusses body image concerns, and provides suggestions for people seeking to achieve weight-related goals. Facts about how physical activity contributes to the success of weight management—and how spending too much time in front of a screen (television, computer, etc.) can disrupt efforts—are also included

Part Six: Eating And Disease explains the link between dietary elements and some specific health conditions, such as heart health and obesity, where food choices may either contribute to, or help prevent, disease. It describes situations where careful adherence to a meal plan is an integral part of disease management strategies, such as avoiding gluten in celiac disease, managing blood sugar in diabetes, and avoiding triggers when food allergies or intolerances are present. The part concludes with information about foodborne illness and eating disorders.

Part Seven: If You Need More Information offers a chapter with cooking tips and suggested resources for finding healthy recipes and planning meals. Directories of dietary and fitness resources are also included.

Bibliographic Note

This volume contains documents and excerpts from publications issued by the following U.S. government agencies: Centers for Disease Control and Prevention (CDC); *Eunice Kennedy Shriver* National Institute of Child Health and Development (NICHD); National Cancer Institute (NCI); National Heart Lung and Blood Institute (NHLBI); National Institute of Allergy and Infectious Diseases (NIAID); National Institute of Arthritis and Musculoskeletal and Skin Diseases (NIAMS); National Institute of Diabetes and Digestive and Kidney Diseases (NIDDK); Office of Disease Prevention and Health Promotion (ODPHP); Office on Dietary Supplements (ODS); Office on Women's Health (OWH); U.S. Department of Agriculture (USDA); U.S. Department of Veterans Affairs (VA); and U.S. Food and Drug Administration (FDA).

In addition, this volume contains copyrighted documents from the following organization: The Nemours Foundation

The photograph on the front cover is © Steve Debenport/iStock.

Medical Review

Omnigraphics contracts with a team of qualified, senior medical professionals who serve as medical consultants for the *Teen Health Series*. As necessary, medical consultants review reprinted and originally written material for currency and accuracy. Citations including the phrase, Reviewed (month, year)" indicate material reviewed by this team. Medical consultation services are provided to the *Teen Health Series* editors by:

Dr. Senthil Selvan, MBBS, DCH, MD
Dr. K. Sivanandham, MBBS, DCH, MS (Research), PhD

About The *Teen Health Series*

At the request of librarians serving today's young adults, the *Teen Health Series* was developed as a specially focused set of volumes within Omnigraphics' *Health Reference Series*. Each volume deals comprehensively with a topic selected according to the needs and interests of people in middle school and high school. Teens seeking preventive guidance, information about disease warning signs, medical statistics, and risk factors for health problems will find answers to their questions in the *Teen Health Series*. The *Series*, however, is not intended to serve as a tool for diagnosing illness, in prescribing treatments, or as a substitute for the physician/patient relationship. All people concerned about medical symptoms or the possibility of disease are encouraged to seek professional care from an appropriate health care provider.

If there is a topic you would like to see addressed in a future volume of the *Teen Health Series*, please write to:

Editor
Teen Health Series
Omnigraphics
615 Griswold, Ste. 901
Detroit, MI 48226

A Note About Spelling And Style

Teen Health Series editors use *Stedman's Medical Dictionary* as an authority for questions related to the spelling of medical terms and the *Chicago Manual of Style* for questions related to grammatical structures, punctuation, and other editorial concerns. Consistent adherence is not always possible, however, because the individual volumes within the *Series* include many documents from a wide variety of different producers and copyright holders, and the editor's primary goal is to present material from each source as accurately as is possible following the terms specified by each document's producer. This sometimes means that information in different chapters or sections may follow other guidelines and alternate spelling authorities.

Part One
Nutrition Fundamentals

Chapter 1
Dietary Guidelines

Dietary Guidelines For Americans At A Glance

Over the past century, deficiencies of essential nutrients have dramatically decreased, many infectious diseases have been conquered, and the majority of the American population can now anticipate a long and productive life. At the same time, rates of chronic diseases—many of which are related to poor quality diet and physical inactivity—have increased. About half of all American adults have one or more preventable, diet-related chronic diseases, including cardiovascular disease, type 2 diabetes, and overweight and obesity.

However, a large body of evidence now shows that healthy eating patterns and regular physical activity can help people achieve and maintain good health and reduce the risk of chronic disease throughout all stages of the lifespan. The *2015–2020 Dietary Guidelines for Americans* (Dietary Guidelines) reflects this evidence through its recommendations.

The Dietary Guidelines is designed for professionals to help all individuals ages two years and older and their families consume a healthy, nutritionally adequate diet. The information in the Dietary Guidelines is used in developing Federal food, nutrition, and health policies and programs. It also is the basis for Federal nutrition education materials designed for the public and for the nutrition education components of U.S. Department of Health and Human Services (HHS) and U.S. Department of Agriculture (USDA) food programs. It is developed for use by policymakers and nutrition and health professionals. Additional audiences who may

About This Chapter: Information in this chapter is excerpted from *"Dietary Guidelines for Americans 2015–2020 Eighth Edition*—Executive Summary," Office of Disease Prevention and Health Promotion (ODPHP), U.S. Department of Health and Human Services (HHS), December 2015.

use Dietary Guidelines information to develop programs, policies, and communication for the general public include businesses, schools, community groups, media, the food industry, and State and local governments.

Previous editions of the Dietary Guidelines focused primarily on individual dietary components such as food groups and nutrients. However, people do not eat food groups and nutrients in isolation but rather in combination, and the totality of the diet forms an overall eating pattern. The components of the eating pattern can have interactive and potentially cumulative effects on health. These patterns can be tailored to an individual's personal preferences, enabling Americans to choose the diet that is right for them. A growing body of research has examined the relationship between overall eating patterns, health, and risk of chronic disease, and findings on these relationships are sufficiently well established to support dietary guidance. As a result, eating patterns and their food and nutrient characteristics are a focus of the recommendations in the Dietary Guidelines.

The Dietary Guidelines provides five overarching guidelines that encourage healthy eating patterns, recognize that individuals will need to make shifts in their food and beverage choices to achieve a healthy pattern, and acknowledge that all segments of our

The Guidelines

1. **Follow a healthy eating pattern across the lifespan.** All food and beverage choices matter. Choose a healthy eating pattern at an appropriate calorie level to help achieve and maintain a healthy body weight, support nutrient adequacy, and reduce the risk of chronic disease.

2. **Focus on variety, nutrient density, and amount.** To meet nutrient needs within calorie limits, choose a variety of nutrient-dense foods across and within all food groups in recommended amounts.

3. **Limit calories from added sugars and saturated fats and reduce sodium intake.** Consume an eating pattern low in added sugars, saturated fats, and sodium. Cut back on foods and beverages higher in these components to amounts that fit within healthy eating patterns.

4. **Shift to healthier food and beverage choices.** Choose nutrient-dense foods and beverages across and within all food groups in place of less healthy choices. Consider cultural and personal preferences to make these shifts easier to accomplish and maintain.

5. **Support healthy eating patterns for all.** Everyone has a role in helping to create and support healthy eating patterns in multiple settings nationwide, from home to school to work to communities.

society have a role to play in supporting healthy choices. These guidelines also embody the idea that a healthy eating pattern is not a rigid prescription, but rather, an adaptable framework in which individuals can enjoy foods that meet their personal, cultural, and traditional preferences and fit within their budget. Several examples of healthy eating patterns that translate and integrate the recommendations in overall healthy ways to eat are provided.

Key Recommendations

The Dietary Guidelines' key recommendations for healthy eating patterns should be applied in their entirety, given the interconnected relationship that each dietary component can have with others.

Consume a healthy eating pattern that accounts for all foods and beverages within an appropriate calorie level.

A healthy eating pattern includes:

- A variety of vegetables from all of the subgroups—dark green, red and orange, legumes (beans and peas), starchy, and other
- Fruits, especially whole fruits
- Grains, at least half of which are whole grains
- Fat-free or low-fat dairy, including milk, yogurt, cheese, and/or fortified soy beverages
- A variety of protein foods, including seafood, lean meats and poultry, eggs, legumes (beans and peas), and nuts, seeds, and soy products
- Oils

A healthy eating pattern limits:

- Saturated fats and *trans* fats, added sugars, and sodium

Key recommendations that are quantitative are provided for several components of the diet that should be limited. These components are of particular public health concern in the United States, and the specified limits can help individuals achieve healthy eating patterns within calorie limits:

- Consume less than 10 percent of calories per day from added sugars
- Consume less than 10 percent of calories per day from saturated fats
- Consume less than 2,300 milligrams (mg) per day of sodium

- If alcohol is consumed, it should be consumed in moderation—up to one drink per day for women and up to two drinks per day for men—and only by adults of legal drinking age.

In tandem with the recommendations above, Americans of all ages—children, adolescents, adults, and older adults—should meet the *Physical Activity Guidelines for Americans* to help promote health and reduce the risk of chronic disease. Americans should aim to achieve and maintain a healthy body weight. The relationship between diet and physical activity contributes to calorie balance and managing body weight.

Chapter 2
Understanding Calories

The Caloric Balance Equation

When it comes to maintaining a healthy weight for a lifetime, the bottom line is—**calories count!** Weight management is all about balance—balancing the number of calories you consume with the number of calories your body uses or "burns off."

- A *calorie* is defined as a unit of energy supplied by food. A calorie is a calorie regardless of its source. Whether you're eating carbohydrates, fats, sugars, or proteins, all of them contain calories.

- *Caloric balance* is like a scale. To remain in balance and maintain your body weight, the calories consumed (from foods) must be balanced by the calories used (in normal body functions, daily activities, and exercise).

Table 2.1. Caloric Balance Status

If you are...	Your caloric balance status is...
Maintaining your weight	"**in balance.**" You are eating roughly the same number of calories that your body is using. Your weight will remain **stable**.
Gaining weight	"**in caloric excess.**" You are eating more calories than your body is using. You will store these extra calories as fat and you'll **gain** weight.
Losing weight	"**in caloric deficit.**" You are eating fewer calories than you are using. Your body is pulling from its fat storage cells for energy, so your weight is **decreasing**.

About This Chapter: Information in this chapter is excerpted from "Healthy Weight," Centers for Disease Control and Prevention (CDC), May 15, 2015.

Am I In Caloric Balance?

If you are maintaining your current body weight, you are in caloric balance. If you need to gain weight or to lose weight, you'll need to tip the balance scale in one direction or another to achieve your goal.

If you need to tip the balance scale in the direction of losing weight, keep in mind that it takes approximately 3,500 calories below your calorie needs to lose a pound of body fat. To lose about 1 to 2 pounds per week, you'll need to reduce your caloric intake by 500—1000 calories per day.

To learn how many calories you are currently eating, begin writing down the foods you eat and the beverages you drink each day. By writing down what you eat and drink, you become more aware of everything you are putting in your mouth. Also, begin writing down the physical activity you do each day and the length of time you do it.

Physical activities (both daily activities and exercise) help tip the balance scale by increasing the calories you expend each day.

Recommended Physical Activity Levels

- 2 hours and 30 minutes (150 minutes) of moderate-intensity aerobic activity (i.e., brisk walking) every week and muscle-strengthening activities on 2 or more days a week that work all major muscle groups (legs, hips, back, abdomen, chest, shoulders, and arms).

- Increasing the intensity or the amount of time that you are physically active can have even greater health benefits and may be needed to control body weight.

The bottom line is… each person's body is unique and may have different caloric needs. A healthy lifestyle requires balance, in the foods you eat, in the beverages you consume, in the way you carry out your daily activities, and in the amount of physical activity or exercise you include in your daily routine. While counting calories is not necessary, it may help you in the beginning to gain an awareness of your eating habits as you strive to achieve energy balance. The ultimate test of balance is whether or not you are gaining, maintaining, or losing weight.

Questions And Answers About Calories

Are Fat-Free And Low-Fat Foods Low In Calories?

Not always. Some fat-free and low-fat foods have extra sugars, which push the calorie amount right back up. Just because a product is fat-free, it doesn't mean that it is "calorie-free." And, calories do count!

Always read the Nutrition Facts food label to find out the calorie content. Remember, this is the calorie content for **one serving** of the food item, so be sure and check the serving size. If you eat more than one serving, you'll be eating more calories than is listed on the food label.

If I Eat Late At Night, Will These Calories Automatically Turn Into Body Fat?

The time of day isn't what affects how your body uses calories. It's the overall number of calories you eat and the calories you burn over the course of 24 hours that affects your weight.

I've Heard It Is More Important To Worry About Carbohydrates Than Calories. Is This True?

By focusing only on carbohydrates, you can still eat too many calories. Also, if you drastically reduce the variety of foods in your diet, you could end up sacrificing vital nutrients and not be able to sustain the diet over time.

Does It Matter How Many Calories I Eat As Long As I'm Maintaining An Active Lifestyle

While physical activity is a vital part of weight control, so is controlling the number of calories you eat. If you consume more calories than you use through normal daily activities and physical activity, you will still gain weight.

What Other Factors Contribute To Overweight And Obesity?

Besides diet and behavior, environment, and genetic factors may also have an effect in causing people to be overweight and obese.

Want to Learn More?

Cutting Calories At Every Meal

You can cut calories by eating foods high in fiber, making better drink choices, avoiding portion size pitfalls, and adding more fruits and vegetables to your eating plan.

Losing Weight

Even a modest weight loss, such as 5 to 10 percent of your total body weight, can produce health benefits.

Physical Activity For A Healthy Weight

Physical activity can increase the number of calories your body uses for energy or "burns off." The burning of calories through physical activity, combined with reducing the number of calories you eat, creates a "calorie deficit" that can help with weight loss.

Chapter 3
Understanding The Food Label

People look at food labels for different reasons. But whatever the reason, many consumers would like to know how to use this information more effectively and easily. The following label-building skills are intended to make it easier for you to use nutrition labels to make quick, informed food choices that contribute to a healthy diet.

Nutrition Facts Panel: An Overview

The information in the main or top section (see #1–4 and #6 on the sample nutrition label below), can vary with each food product; it contains product-specific information (serving size, calories, and nutrient information). The bottom part (see #5 on the sample label below) contains a footnote with Daily Values (DVs) for 2,000 and 2,500 calorie diets. This footnote provides recommended dietary information for important nutrients, including fats, sodium and fiber. The footnote is found only on larger packages and does not change from product to product.

The Serving Size

(#1 in Figure 3.1)

The first place to start when you look at the Nutrition Facts label is the serving size and the number of servings in the package. Serving sizes are standardized to make it easier to compare similar foods; they are provided in familiar units, such as cups or pieces, followed by the metric amount, e.g., the number of grams.

About This Chapter: Information in this chapter is excerpted from "How to Understand and Use the Nutrition Facts Label," U.S. Food and Drug Administration (FDA), May 25, 2016.

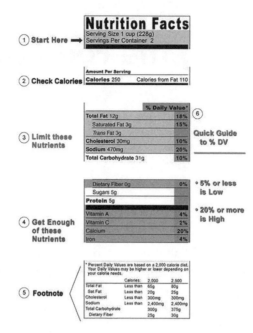

Figure 3.1. Sample Label For Macaroni And Cheese

The size of the serving on the food package influences the number of calories and all the nutrient amounts listed on the top part of the label. **Pay attention to the serving size, especially how many servings there are in the food package. Then ask yourself, "How many servings am I consuming"? (e.g., 1/2 serving, 1 serving, or more)** In the sample label, one serving of macaroni and cheese equals one cup. If you ate the whole package, you would eat **two** cups. That doubles the calories and other nutrient numbers, including the %Daily Values as shown in the sample label.

Table 3.1. The Serving Size (An Example)

	Single Serving	**%DV**	**Double Serving**	**%DV**
Serving Size	1 cup (228g)		2 cups (456g)	
Calories	250		500	
Calories from Fat	110		220	
Total Fat	12g	18%	24g	36%
Trans Fat	1.5g		3g	
Saturated Fat	3g	15%	6g	30%

Table 3.1. Continued

	Single Serving	%DV	Double Serving	%DV
Cholesterol	30mg	10%	60mg	20%
Sodium	470mg	20%	940mg	40%
Total Carbohydrate	31g	10%	62g	20%
Dietary Fiber	0g	0%	0g	0%
Sugars	5g		10g	
Protein	5g		10g	
Vitamin A		4%		8%
Vitamin C		2%		4%
Calcium		20%		40%
Iron		4%		8%

Calories (And Calories From Fat)

Calories provide a measure of how much energy you get from a serving of this food. Many Americans consume more calories than they need without meeting recommended intakes for a number of nutrients. The calorie section of the label can help you manage your weight (i.e., gain, lose, or maintain.)

Remember: the number of servings you consume determines the number of calories you actually eat (your portion amount).

(#2 in Figure 3.1)

In the example, there are 250 calories in one serving of this macaroni and cheese. How many calories from fat are there in ONE serving? Answer: 110 calories, which means almost half the calories in a single serving come from fat. What if you ate the whole package content? Then, you would consume two servings, or 500 calories, and 220 would come from fat.

General Guide To Calories

- 40 Calories is low

- 100 Calories is moderate

- 400 Calories or more is high

The General Guide to Calories provides a general reference for calories when you look at a Nutrition Facts label. This guide is based on a 2,000 calorie diet.

Eating too many calories per day is linked to overweight and obesity.

The Nutrients: How Much?

Look at the top of the nutrient section in the sample label. It shows you some key nutrients that impact on your health and separates them into two main groups:

Limit These Nutrients

(#3 in Figure 3.1)

Total Fat 12g	18%
Saturated Fat 3g	15%
Trans Fat 3g	
Cholesterol 30mg	10%
Sodium 470mg	20%

Figure 3.2. Limit These Nutrients

The nutrients listed first are the ones Americans generally eat in adequate amounts, or even too much. Eating too much fat, saturated fat, *trans* fat, cholesterol, or sodium may increase your risk of certain chronic diseases, like heart disease, some cancers, or high blood pressure.

Important: Health experts recommend that you keep your intake of saturated fat, *trans* fat and cholesterol as low as possible as part of a nutritionally balanced diet.

Get Enough Of These

(#4 in Figure 3.1)

Most Americans don't get enough dietary fiber, vitamin A, vitamin C, calcium, and iron in their diets. Eating enough of these nutrients can improve your health and help reduce the risk of some diseases and conditions. For example, getting enough calcium may reduce the risk of osteoporosis, a condition that results in brittle bones as one ages. Eating a diet high in dietary fiber promotes healthy bowel function. Additionally, a diet rich in fruits, vegetables, and grain

Dietary Fiber 0g	0%
Vitamin A	4%
Vitamin C	2%
Calcium	20%
Iron	4%

Figure 3.3. Get Enough Of These

products that contain dietary fiber, particularly soluble fiber, and low in saturated fat and cholesterol may reduce the risk of heart disease.

Remember: You can use the Nutrition Facts label not only to help limit those nutrients you want to cut back on but also to *increase* those nutrients you need to consume in greater amounts.

Understanding The Footnote On The Bottom Of The Nutrition Facts Label

(#5 in Figure 3.1)

*Percent Daily Values are based on a 2,000 calorie diet. Your Daily Values may be higher or lower depending on your calorie needs.	Calories:	2,000	2,500
Total Fat	Less than	65g	80g
Sat Fat	Less than	20g	25g
Cholesterol	Less than	300mg	300mg
Sodium	Less than	2,400mg	2,400mg
Total Carbohydrate		300g	375g
Dietary Fiber		25g	30g

Figure 3.4. Daily Values (DV)

Note the * used after the heading "%Daily Value" on the Nutrition Facts label. It refers to the Footnote in the lower part of the nutrition label, which tells you "**%DVs are based on a 2,000 calorie diet.**" This statement must be on all food labels. But the remaining information in the full footnote may not be on the package if the size of the label is too small. When the full footnote does appear, it will always be the same. It doesn't change from product to product, because it shows recommended dietary advice for all Americans—it is not about a specific food product.

Look at the amounts circled in the footnote—these are the Daily Values (DVs) for each nutrient listed and are based on public health experts' advice. DVs are recommended levels of intakes. DVs in the footnote are based on a 2,000 or 2,500 calorie diet. Note how the DVs for some nutrients change, while others (for cholesterol and sodium) remain the same for both calorie amounts.

How The DVs Relate To The %DVs

Look at the example below for another way to see how the DVs relate to the %DVs and dietary guidance. For each nutrient listed there is a DV, a %DV, and dietary advice or a goal. If you follow this dietary advice, you will stay within public health experts' recommended upper or lower limits for the nutrients listed, based on a 2,000 calorie daily diet.

Examples Of DVs Versus %DVs

Table 3.2. Based on A 2,000 Calorie Diet

Nutrient	DV	%DV	Goal
Total Fat	65g	= 100%DV	Less than
Sat Fat	20g	= 100%DV	Less than
Cholesterol	300mg	= 100%DV	Less than
Sodium	2400mg	= 100%DV	Less than
Total Carbohydrate	300g	= 100%DV	At least
Dietary Fiber	25g	= 100%DV	At least

Upper Limit—Eat "Less Than"

The nutrients that have "upper daily limits" are listed first on the footnote of larger labels and on the example above. Upper limits means it is recommended that you stay below—eat "less than"—the Daily Value nutrient amounts listed per day. For example, the DV for Saturated fat is 20g. This amount is 100%DV for this nutrient. What is the goal or dietary advice? To eat "less than" 20 g or 100%DV for the day.

Lower Limit—Eat "At Least"

Now look at the section where dietary fiber is listed. The DV for dietary fiber is 25g, which is 100% DV. This means it is recommended that you eat "at least" this amount of dietary fiber per day.

The DV for Total Carbohydrate (section in white) is 300g or 100%DV. This amount is recommended for a balanced daily diet that is based on 2,000 calories, but can vary, depending on your daily intake of fat and protein.

The Percent Daily Value (%DV)

The % Daily Values (%DVs) are based on the Daily Value recommendations for key nutrients but only for a 2,000 calorie daily diet—not 2,500 calories. You, like most people, may not know how many calories you consume in a day. But you can still use the %DV as a frame of reference whether or not you consume more or less than 2,000 calories.

The %DV helps you determine if a serving of food is high or low in a nutrient. Note: a few nutrients, like *trans* fat, do not have a %DV.

Do you need to know how to calculate percentages to use the %DV? No, the label (the %DV) does the math for you. It helps you interpret the numbers (grams and milligrams) by putting them all on the same scale for the day (0–100%DV). The %DV column doesn't add up vertically to 100%. Instead each nutrient is based on 100% of the daily requirements for that nutrient (for a 2,000 calorie diet). This way you can tell high from low and know which nutrients contribute a lot, or a little, to your **daily** recommended allowance (upper or lower).

Quick Guide To %DV

5%DV or less is low and 20%DV or more is high

(#6 in Figure 3.1)

This guide tells you that **5%DV or less is low** for all nutrients, those you want to limit (e.g., fat, saturated fat, cholesterol, and sodium), or for those that you want to consume in greater amounts (fiber, calcium, etc). As the **Quick Guide** shows, **20%DV or more is high** for all nutrients.

Example: Look at the amount of Total Fat in one serving listed on the sample nutrition label. Is 18%DV contributing a lot or a little to your fat limit of 100%DV? Check the **Quick Guide to %DV**. 18%DV, which is below 20%DV, is not yet high, but what if you ate the whole package (two servings)? You would double that amount, eating 36 percent of your daily allowance for Total Fat. Coming from just one food, that amount leaves you with 64 percent of your fat allowance (100%–36%=64%) for *all* of the other foods you eat that day, snacks and drinks included.

	% Daily Value*
Total Fat 12g	18%
Saturated Fat 3g	15%
Trans Fat 3g	
Cholesterol 30mg	10%
Sodium 470mg	20%
Total Carbohydrate 31g	10%
Dietary Fiber 0g	0%
Sugars 5g	
Protein 5g	
Vitamin A	4%
Vitamin C	2%
Calcium	20%
Iron	4%

Figure 3.5. Quick Guide To %DV

Using The %DV

Comparisons: The %DV also makes it easy for you to make comparisons. You can compare one product or brand to a similar product. Just make sure the serving sizes are similar, especially the weight (e.g., gram, milligram, ounces) of each product. It's easy to see which foods are higher or lower in nutrients because the serving sizes are generally consistent for similar types of foods, except in a few cases like cereals.

Nutrient Content Claims: Use the %DV to help you quickly distinguish one claim from another, such as "reduced fat" vs. "light" or "nonfat." Just compare the %DVs for Total Fat in each food product to see which one is higher or lower in that nutrient—there is no need to memorize definitions. This works when comparing all nutrient content claims, e.g., less, light, low, free, more, high, etc.

Dietary Trade-Offs: You can use the %DV to help you make dietary trade-offs with other foods throughout the day. You don't have to give up a favorite food to eat a healthy diet. When a food you like is high in fat, balance it with foods that are low in fat at other times of the day. Also, pay attention to how much you eat so that the total amount of fat for the day stays below 100%DV.

Nutrients With A %DV But No Weight Listed—Spotlight On Calcium

Serving Size 1 cup (236ml)	
Servings Per Container 1	

Amount Per Serving	
Calories 80	Calories from Fat 0

	% Daily Value*
Total Fat 0g	0%
Saturated Fat 0g	0%
Trans Fat 0g	
Cholesterol Less than 5mg	0%
Sodium 120mg	5%
Total Carbohydrate 11g	4%
Dietary Fiber 0g	0%
Sugars 11g	
Protein 9g	17%

Vitamin A 10%	•	Vitamin C 4%
Calcium 30% • Iron 0% • Vitamin D 25%		

*Percent Daily Values are based on a 2,000 calorie diet. Your daily values may be higher or lower depending on your calorie needs.

Figure 3.6. Nutrition Facts

Calcium: Look at the %DV for calcium on food packages so you know how much one serving contributes to the *total amount you need* per day. Remember, a food with 20%DV or more contributes a lot of calcium to your daily total, while one with 5%DV or less contributes a little.

Experts advise adult consumers to consume adequate amounts of calcium, that is, 1,000mg or 100%DV in a daily 2,000 calorie diet. This advice is often given in milligrams (mg), but the Nutrition Facts label **only** lists a %DV for calcium.

For certain populations, they advise that adolescents, especially girls, consume 1,300mg (130%DV) and post-menopausal women consume 1,200mg (120%DV) of calcium daily. The DV for calcium on food labels is 1,000mg.

Don't be fooled—always check the label for calcium because you can't make assumptions about the amount of calcium in specific food categories. Example: the amount of calcium in milk, whether skim or whole, is generally the same per serving, whereas the amount of calcium in the same size yogurt container (8oz) can vary from 20–45 %DV.

Nutrients Without A %DV: Trans Fats, Protein, And Sugars

Note that *Trans* fat, Sugars and, Protein do not list a %DV on the Nutrition Facts label.

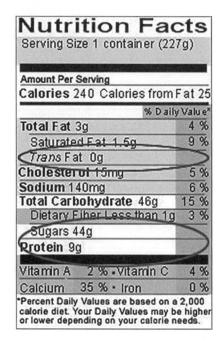

Figure 3.7. Plain Yogurt   **Figure 3.8.** Fruit Yogurt

Trans Fat: Experts could not provide a reference value for *trans* fat nor any other information that U.S. Food and Drug Administration (FDA) believes is sufficient to establish a Daily Value or %DV. Scientific reports link *trans* fat (and saturated fat) with raising blood LDL ("bad") cholesterol levels, both of which increase your risk of coronary heart disease, a leading cause of death in the United States.

> **Important:** Health experts recommend that you keep your intake of saturated fat, *trans* fat and cholesterol as low as possible as part of a nutritionally balanced diet.

Protein: A %DV is required to be listed if a claim is made for protein, such as "high in protein." Otherwise, unless the food is meant for use by infants and children under 4 years old, none is needed. Current scientific evidence indicates that protein intake is not a public health concern for adults and children over 4 years of age.

Sugars: No daily reference value has been established for sugars because no recommendations have been made for the total amount to eat in a day. Keep in mind, the sugars listed on the Nutrition Facts label include naturally occurring sugars (like those in fruit and milk) as well as those added to a food or drink. Check the ingredient list for specifics on added sugars.

Take a look at the Nutrition Facts label for the two yogurt examples. The plain yogurt on the left has 10g of sugars, while the fruit yogurt on the right has 44g of sugars in one serving.

Now look below at the ingredient lists for the two yogurts. Ingredients are listed in descending order of weight (from most to least). Note that no added sugars or sweeteners are in the list of ingredients for the plain yogurt, yet 10g of sugars were listed on the Nutrition Facts label. This is because there are no added sugars in plain yogurt, only naturally occurring sugars (lactose in the milk).

Plain Yogurt—contains no added sugars

> INGREDIENTS: CULTURED PASTEURIZED GRADE A NONFAT MILK, WHEY PROTEIN CONCENTRATE, PECTIN, CARRAGEENAN.

Figure 3.9. Ingredients For Plain Yogurt

Fruit Yogurt—contains added sugars

> INGREDIENTS: CULTURED GRADE A REDUCED FAT MILK, APPLES, HIGH FRUCTOSE CORN SYRUP, CINNAMON, NUTMEG, NATURAL FLAVORS, AND PECTIN. CONTAINS ACTIVE YOGURT AND L. ACIDOPHILUS CULTURES.

Figure 3.10. Ingredients For Fruit Yogurt

If you are concerned about your intake of sugars, make sure that added sugars are not listed as one of the first few ingredients. Other names for added sugars include: corn syrup, high-fructose corn syrup, fruit juice concentrate, maltose, dextrose, sucrose, honey, and maple syrup.

To limit nutrients that have no %DV, like *trans* fat and sugars, compare the labels of similar products and choose the food with the lowest amount.

Chapter 4
Grains

What Foods Are In The Grains Group?

Any food made from wheat, rice, oats, cornmeal, barley or another cereal grain is a grain product. Bread, pasta, oatmeal, breakfast cereals, tortillas, and grits are examples of grain products.

Grains are divided into 2 subgroups, Whole Grains and Refined Grains. Whole grains contain the entire grain kernel, the bran, germ, and endosperm. Examples of whole grains include whole-wheat flour, bulgur (cracked wheat), oatmeal, whole cornmeal, and brown rice. Refined grains have been milled, a process that removes the bran and germ. This is done to give grains a finer texture and improve their shelf life, but it also removes dietary fiber, iron, and many B vitamins. *Some examples of refined grain products* are white flour, de-germed cornmeal, white bread, and white rice.

Most refined grains are enriched. This means certain B vitamins (thiamin, riboflavin, niacin, folic acid) and iron are added back after processing. Fiber is not added back to enriched grains. Check the ingredient list on refined grain products to make sure that the word "enriched" is included in the grain name. Some food products are made from mixtures of whole grains and refined grains.

About This Chapter: Information in this chapter is excerpted from "All about the Grains Group," U.S. Department of Agriculture (USDA), July 26, 2016.

How Many Grain Foods Are Needed Daily?

The amount of grains you need to eat depends on your age, sex, and level of physical activity. Recommended daily amounts are listed in this table below. Most Americans consume enough grains, but few are whole grains. **At least half of all the grains eaten should be whole grains.**

Table 4.1. Daily Grain Table

		Daily Recommendation*	Daily minimum amount of whole grains
Girls	9–13 years old	5 ounce equivalents	3 ounce equivalents
	14–18 years old	6 ounce equivalents	3 ounce equivalents
Boys	9–13 years old	6 ounce equivalents	3 ounce equivalents
	14–18 years old	8 ounce equivalents	4 ounce equivalents

*These amounts are appropriate for individuals who get less than 30 minutes per day of moderate physical activity, beyond normal daily activities. Those who are more physically active may be able to consume more while staying within calorie needs.

What Counts As An Ounce-Equivalent Of Grains?

In general, 1 slice of bread, 1 cup of ready-to-eat cereal, or ½ cup of cooked rice, cooked pasta, or cooked cereal can be considered as 1 ounce-equivalent from the Grains Group.

Why Is It Important To Eat Grains, Especially Whole Grains?

Eating grains, especially whole grains, provides health benefits. People who eat whole grains as part of a healthy diet have a reduced risk of some chronic diseases. Grains provide many nutrients that are vital for the health and maintenance of our bodies.

Nutrients

- Grains are important sources of many nutrients, including dietary fiber, several B vitamins (thiamin, riboflavin, niacin, and folate), and minerals (iron, magnesium, and selenium).

- Dietary fiber from whole grains or other foods, may help reduce blood cholesterol levels and may lower risk of heart disease, obesity, and type 2 diabetes. Fiber is important for proper bowel function. It helps reduce constipation and diverticulosis. Fiber-containing foods such as whole grains help provide a feeling of fullness with fewer calories.

- The B vitamins thiamin, riboflavin, and niacin play a key role in metabolism–they help the body release energy from protein, fat, and carbohydrates. B vitamins are also essential for a healthy nervous system. Many refined grains are enriched with these B vitamins.

- Folate (folic acid), another B vitamin, helps the body form red blood cells. Women of childbearing age who may become pregnant should consume adequate folate from foods, and in addition 400 mcg of synthetic folic acid from fortified foods or supplements. This reduces the risk of neural tube defects, spina bifida, and anencephaly during fetal development.

- Iron is used to carry oxygen in the blood. Many teenage girls and women in their childbearing years have iron-deficiency anemia. They should eat foods high in heme iron (meats) or eat other iron containing foods along with foods rich in vitamin C, which can improve absorption of non-heme iron. Whole and enriched refined grain products are major sources of non-heme iron in American diets.

- Whole grains are sources of magnesium and selenium. Magnesium is a mineral used in building bones and releasing energy from muscles. Selenium protects cells from oxidation. It is also important for a healthy immune system.

Health Benefits

- Consuming whole grains as part of a healthy diet may reduce the risk of heart disease.

- Consuming foods containing fiber, such as whole grains, as part of a healthy diet, may reduce constipation.

- Eating whole grains may help with weight management.

- Eating grain products fortified with folate before and during pregnancy helps prevent neural tube defects during fetal development.

Tips To Help You Eat Whole Grains
At Meals

- To eat more whole grains, substitute a whole-grain product for a refined product—such as eating whole-wheat bread instead of white bread or brown rice instead of white rice. It's important to *substitute* the whole-grain product for the refined one, rather than *adding* the whole-grain product.

- For a change, try brown rice or whole-wheat pasta. Try brown rice stuffing in baked green peppers or tomatoes and whole-wheat macaroni in macaroni and cheese.

- Use whole grains in mixed dishes, such as barley in vegetable soup or stews and bulgur wheat in a casserole or stir-fry.

- Create a whole grain pilaf with a mixture of barley, wild rice, brown rice, broth and spices. For a special touch, stir in toasted nuts or chopped dried fruit.

- Experiment by substituting whole wheat or oat flour for up to half of the flour in pancake, waffle, muffin or other flour-based recipes. They may need a bit more leavening.

- Use whole-grain bread or cracker crumbs in meatloaf.

- Try rolled oats or a crushed, unsweetened whole grain cereal as breading for baked chicken, fish, veal cutlets, or eggplant parmesan.

- Try an unsweetened, whole grain ready-to-eat cereal as croutons in salad or in place of crackers with soup.

- Freeze leftover cooked brown rice, bulgur, or barley. Heat and serve it later as a quick side dish.

As Snacks

- Snack on ready-to-eat, whole grain cereals such as toasted oat cereal.

- Add whole-grain flour or oatmeal when making cookies or other baked treats.

- Try 100 percent whole-grain snack crackers.

- Popcorn, a whole grain, can be a healthy snack if made with little or no added salt and butter.

What To Look For On The Food Label

- Choose foods that name one of the following whole-grain ingredients first on the label's ingredient list:

Whole Grain Ingredients

- brown rice
- buckwheat
- bulgur

- millet
- oatmeal
- popcorn

- quinoa
- rolled oats
- whole-grain barley
- whole-grain corn
- whole-grain sorghum
- whole-grain triticale
- whole oats
- whole rye
- whole wheat
- wild rice

- Foods labeled with the words "multi-grain," "stone-ground," "100% wheat," "cracked wheat," "seven-grain," or "bran" are usually not whole-grain products.

- Color is not an indication of a whole grain. Bread can be brown because of molasses or other added ingredients. Read the ingredient list to see if it is a whole grain.

- Use the Nutrition Facts label and choose whole grain products with a higher % Daily Value (%DV) for fiber. Many, but not all, whole grain products are good or excellent sources of fiber.

- Read the food label's ingredient list. Look for terms that indicate added sugars (such as sucrose, high-fructose corn syrup, honey, malt syrup, maple syrup, molasses, or raw sugar) that add extra calories. Choose foods with fewer added sugars.

- Most sodium in the food supply comes from packaged foods. Similar packaged foods can vary widely in sodium content, including breads. Use the Nutrition Facts label to choose foods with a lower %DV for sodium. Foods with less than 140 mg sodium per serving can be labeled as low sodium foods. Claims such as "low in sodium" or "very low in sodium" on the front of the food label can help you identify foods that contain less salt (or sodium).

Chapter 5
Vegetables

What Foods Are In The Vegetable Group?

Any vegetable or 100 percent vegetable juice counts as a member of the Vegetable Group. Vegetables may be raw or cooked; fresh, frozen, canned or dried/dehydrated; and may be whole, cut-up or mashed.

Based on their nutrient content, vegetables are organized into five subgroups: dark-green vegetables, starchy vegetables, red and orange vegetables, beans and peas, and other vegetables.

How Many Vegetables Are Needed?

The amount of vegetables you need to eat depends on your age, sex, and level of physical activity. Recommended total daily amounts and recommended weekly amounts from each vegetable subgroup are shown in the two tables below.

Table 5.1. Daily Vegetable Table

Daily Recommendation*		
Girls	9–13 years old	2 cups
	14–18 years old	2 ½ cups
Boys	9–13 years old	2 ½ cups
	14–18 years old	3 cups

*These amounts are appropriate for individuals who get less than 30 minutes per day of moderate physical activity, beyond normal daily activities. Those who are more physically active may be able to consume more while staying within calorie needs.

About This Chapter: Information in this chapter is excerpted from "All about the Vegetable Group," ChooseMyPlate.gov, U.S. Department of Agriculture (USDA), July 26, 2016.

Vegetable subgroup recommendations are given as amounts to eat WEEKLY. It is not necessary to eat vegetables from each subgroup daily. However, over a week, try to consume the amounts listed from each subgroup as a way to reach your daily intake recommendation.

Table 5.2. Weekly Vegetable Subgroup Table

	Dark green vegetables	Red and orange vegetables	Beans and peas	Starchy vegetables	Other vegetables
	Amount per Week				
Girls					
9–13 yrs old	1 ½ cups	4 cups	1 cup	4 cups	3 ½ cups
14–18 yrs old	1 ½ cups	5 ½ cups	1 ½ cups	5 cups	4 cups
Boys					
9–13 yrs old	1 ½ cups	5 ½ cups	1 ½ cups	5 cups	4 cups
14–18 yrs old	2 cups	6 cups	2 cups	6 cups	5 cups

What Counts As A Cup Of Vegetables?

In general, 1 cup of raw or cooked vegetables or vegetable juice or 2 cups of raw leafy greens can be considered as 1 cup from the Vegetable Group.

Why Is It Important To Eat Vegetables?

Eating vegetables provides health benefits—people who eat more vegetables and fruits as part of an overall healthy diet are likely to have a reduced risk of some chronic diseases. Vegetables provide nutrients vital for health and maintenance of your body.

Nutrients

- Most vegetables are naturally low in fat and calories. None have cholesterol. (Sauces or seasonings may add fat, calories, and/or cholesterol.)

- Vegetables are important sources of many nutrients, including potassium, dietary fiber, folate (folic acid), vitamin A, and vitamin C.

- Diets rich in potassium may help to maintain healthy blood pressure. Vegetable sources of potassium include sweet potatoes, white potatoes, white beans, tomato products (paste, sauce, and juice), beet greens, soybeans, lima beans, spinach, lentils, and kidney beans.

- Dietary fiber from vegetables, as part of an overall healthy diet, helps reduce blood cholesterol levels and may lower risk of heart disease. Fiber is important for proper bowel function. It helps reduce constipation and diverticulosis. Fiber-containing foods such as vegetables help provide a feeling of fullness with fewer calories.

- Folate (folic acid) helps the body form red blood cells. Women of childbearing age who may become pregnant should consume adequate folate from foods, and in addition 400 mcg of synthetic folic acid from fortified foods or supplements. This reduces the risk of neural tube defects, spina bifida, and anencephaly during fetal development.

- Vitamin A keeps eyes and skin healthy and helps to protect against infections.

- Vitamin C helps heal cuts and wounds and keeps teeth and gums healthy. Vitamin C aids in iron absorption.

Health Benefits

- Eating a diet rich in vegetables and fruits as part of an overall healthy diet may reduce risk for heart disease, including heart attack and stroke.

- Eating a diet rich in some vegetables and fruits as part of an overall healthy diet may protect against certain types of cancers.

- Diets rich in foods containing fiber, such as some vegetables and fruits, may reduce the risk of heart disease, obesity, and type 2 diabetes.

- Eating vegetables and fruits rich in potassium as part of an overall healthy diet may lower blood pressure, and may also reduce the risk of developing kidney stones and help to decrease bone loss.

- Eating foods such as vegetables that are lower in calories per cup instead of some other higher-calorie food may be useful in helping to lower calorie intake.

Tips To Help You Eat Vegetables

In General

- Buy fresh vegetables in season. They cost less and are likely to be at their peak flavor.

- Stock up on frozen vegetables for quick and easy cooking in the microwave.

- Buy vegetables that arc easy to prepare. Pick up pre-washed bags of salad greens and add baby carrots or grape tomatoes for a salad in minutes. Buy packages of veggies such as baby carrots or celery sticks for quick snacks.

- Use a microwave to quickly "zap" vegetables. White or sweet potatoes can be baked quickly this way.

- Vary your veggie choices to keep meals interesting.

- Try crunchy vegetables, raw or lightly steamed.

For The Best Nutritional Value

- Select vegetables with more potassium often, such as sweet potatoes, white potatoes, white beans, tomato products (paste, sauce, and juice), beet greens, soybeans, lima beans, spinach, lentils, and kidney beans.

- Sauces or seasonings can add calories, saturated fat, and sodium to vegetables. Use the Nutrition Facts label to compare the calories and % Daily Value for saturated fat and sodium in plain and seasoned vegetables.

- Prepare more foods from fresh ingredients to lower sodium intake. Most sodium in the food supply comes from packaged or processed foods.

- Buy canned vegetables labeled "reduced sodium," "low sodium," or "no salt added." If you want to add a little salt it will likely be less than the amount in the regular canned product.

At Meals

- Plan some meals around a vegetable main dish, such as a vegetable stir-fry or soup. Then add other foods to complement it.

- Try a main dish salad for lunch. Go light on the salad dressing.

- Include a green salad with your dinner every night.

- Shred carrots or zucchini into meatloaf, casseroles, quick breads, and muffins.

- Include chopped vegetables in pasta sauce or lasagna.

- Order a veggie pizza with toppings like mushrooms, green peppers, and onions, and ask for extra veggies.

- Use pureed, cooked vegetables such as potatoes to thicken stews, soups, and gravies. These add flavor, nutrients, and texture.

- Grill vegetable kabobs as part of a barbecue meal. Try tomatoes, mushrooms, green peppers, and onions.

Make Vegetables More Appealing

- Many vegetables taste great with a dip or dressing. Try a low-fat salad dressing with raw broccoli, red and green peppers, celery sticks or cauliflower.

- Add color to salads by adding baby carrots, shredded red cabbage or spinach leaves. Include in-season vegetables for variety through the year.

- Include beans or peas in flavorful mixed dishes, such as chili or minestrone soup.

- Decorate plates or serving dishes with vegetable slices.

- Keep a bowl of cut-up vegetables in a see-through container in the refrigerator. Carrot and celery sticks are traditional, but consider red or green pepper strips, broccoli florets or cucumber slices.

Keep It Safe

- Rinse vegetables before preparing or eating them. Under clean, running water, rub vegetables briskly with your hands to remove dirt and surface microorganisms. Dry with a clean cloth towel or paper towel after rinsing.

- Keep vegetables separate from raw meat, poultry and seafood while shopping, preparing or storing.

Chapter 6
Fruits

What Foods Are In The Fruit Group?

Any fruit or 100 percent fruit juice counts as part of the Fruit Group. Fruits may be fresh, canned, frozen or dried, and may be whole, cut-up or pureed.

How Much Fruit Is Needed Daily?

The amount of fruit you need to eat depends on age, sex, and level of physical activity. Recommended daily amounts are shown in the table below.

Table 6.1. Daily Fruit Table

Daily Recommendation*		
Girls	9–13 years old	1 ½ cups
	14–18 years old	1 ½ cups
Boys	9–13 years old	1 ½ cups
	14–18 years old	2 cups

*These amounts are appropriate for individuals who get less than 30 minutes per day of moderate physical activity, beyond normal daily activities. Those who are more physically active may be able to consume more while staying within calorie needs.

About This Chapter: Information in this chapter is excerpted from "All about the Fruit Group," ChooseMyPlate.gov, U.S. Department of Agriculture (USDA), July 26, 2016.

What Counts As A Cup Of Fruit?

In general, 1 cup of fruit or 100 percent fruit juice or ½ cup of dried fruit can be considered as 1 cup from the Fruit Group.

Why Is It Important To Eat Fruit?

Eating fruit provides health benefits—people who eat more fruits and vegetables as part of an overall healthy diet are likely to have a reduced risk of some chronic diseases. Fruits provide nutrients vital for health and maintenance of your body.

Nutrients

- Most fruits are naturally low in fat, sodium, and calories. None have cholesterol.

- Fruits are sources of many essential nutrients that are under consumed, including potassium, dietary fiber, vitamin C, and folate (folic acid).

- Diets rich in potassium may help to maintain healthy blood pressure. Fruit sources of potassium include bananas, prunes and prune juice, dried peaches and apricots, cantaloupe, honeydew melon, and orange juice.

- Dietary fiber from fruits, as part of an overall healthy diet, helps reduce blood cholesterol levels and may lower risk of heart disease. Fiber is important for proper bowel function. It helps reduce constipation and diverticulosis. Fiber-containing foods such as fruits help provide a feeling of fullness with fewer calories. Whole or cut-up fruits are sources of dietary fiber; fruit juices contain little or no fiber.

- Vitamin C is important for growth and repair of all body tissues, helps heal cuts and wounds, and keeps teeth and gums healthy.

- Folate (folic acid) helps the body form red blood cells. Women of childbearing age who may become pregnant should consume adequate folate from foods, and in addition 400 mcg of synthetic folic acid from fortified foods or supplements. This reduces the risk of neural tube defects, spina bifida, and anencephaly during fetal development.

Health Benefits

- Eating a diet rich in vegetables and fruits as part of an overall healthy diet may reduce risk for heart disease, including heart attack and stroke.

- Eating a diet rich in some vegetables and fruits as part of an overall healthy diet may protect against certain types of cancers.

- Diets rich in foods containing fiber, such as some vegetables and fruits, may reduce the risk of heart disease, obesity, and type 2 diabetes.

- Eating vegetables and fruits rich in potassium as part of an overall healthy diet may lower blood pressure, and may also reduce the risk of developing kidney stones and help to decrease bone loss.

- Eating foods such as fruits that are lower in calories per cup instead of some other higher-calorie food may be useful in helping to lower calorie intake.

Tips To Help You Eat Fruits

In General

- Keep a bowl of whole fruit on the table, counter or in the refrigerator.

- Refrigerate cut-up fruit to store for later.

- Buy fresh fruits in season when they may be less expensive and at their peak flavor.

- Buy fruits that are dried, frozen, and canned (in water or 100 percent juice) as well as fresh, so that you always have a supply on hand.

- Consider convenience when shopping. Try pre-cut packages of fruit (such as melon or pineapple chunks) for a healthy snack in seconds. Choose packaged fruits that do not have added sugars.

For The Best Nutritional Value

- Make most of your choices whole or cut-up fruit rather than juice, for the benefits dietary fiber provides.

- Select fruits with more potassium often, such as bananas, prunes and prune juice, dried peaches and apricots, and orange juice.

- When choosing canned fruits, select fruit canned in 100 percent fruit juice or water rather than syrup.

- Vary your fruit choices. Fruits differ in nutrient content.

At Meals

- At breakfast, top your cereal with bananas or peaches; add blueberries to pancakes; drink 100 percent orange or grapefruit juice. Or, mix fresh fruit with plain fat-free or low-fat yogurt.

- At lunch, pack a tangerine, banana or grapes to eat or choose fruits from a salad bar. Individual containers of fruits like peaches or applesauce are easy and convenient.

- At dinner, add crushed pineapple to coleslaw or include orange sections or grapes in a tossed salad.

- Make a Waldorf salad, with apples, celery, walnuts, and a low-calorie salad dressing.

- Try meat dishes that incorporate fruit, such as chicken with apricots or mangoes.

- Add fruit like pineapple or peaches to kabobs as part of a barbecue meal.

- For dessert, have baked apples, pears or a fruit salad.

As Snacks

- Cut-up fruit makes a great snack. Either cut them yourself or buy pre-cut packages of fruit pieces like pineapples or melons. Or, try whole fresh berries or grapes.

- Dried fruits also make a great snack. They are easy to carry and store well. Because they are dried, ¼ cup is equivalent to ½ cup of other fruits.

- Keep a package of dried fruit in your desk or bag. Some fruits that are available dried include apricots, apples, pineapple, bananas, cherries, figs, dates, cranberries, blueberries, prunes (dried plums), and raisins (dried grapes).

- As a snack, spread peanut butter on apple slices or top plain fat-free or low-fat yogurt with berries or slices of kiwi fruit.

- Frozen juice bars (100% juice) make healthy alternatives to high-fat snacks.

Make Fruit More Appealing

- Many fruits taste great with a dip or dressing. Try fat-free or low-fat yogurt as a dip for fruits like strawberries or melons.

- Make a fruit smoothie by blending fat-free or low-fat milk or yogurt with fresh or frozen fruit. Try bananas, peaches, strawberries or other berries.

- Try unsweetened applesauce as a lower calorie substitute for some of the oil when baking cakes.

- Try different textures of fruits. For example, apples are crunchy, bananas are smooth and creamy, and oranges are juicy.

- For fresh fruit salads, mix apples, bananas or pears with acidic fruits like oranges, pineapple or lemon juice to keep them from turning brown.

Keep It Safe

- Rinse fruits before preparing or eating them. Under clean, running water, rub fruits briskly with your hands to remove dirt and surface microorganisms. Dry with a clean cloth towel or paper towel after rinsing.
- Keep fruits separate from raw meat, poultry and seafood while shopping, preparing or storing.

Chapter 7
The Dairy Group

What Foods Are Included In The Dairy Group?

All fluid milk products and many foods made from milk are considered part of this food group. Most Dairy Group choices should be fat-free or low-fat. Foods made from milk that retain their calcium content are part of the group. Foods made from milk that have little to no calcium, such as cream cheese, cream, and butter, are not. Calcium-fortified soymilk (soy beverage) is also part of the Dairy Group.

How Much Food From The Dairy Group Is Needed Daily?

The amount of food from the Dairy Group you need to eat depends on age. Recommended daily amounts are shown in the table below.

Table 7.1. Daily Dairy Table

Daily Recommendation

Girls	9–13 years old	3 cups
	14–18 years old	3 cups
Boys	9–13 years old	3 cups
	14–18 years old	3 cups

About This Chapter: Information in this chapter is excerpted from "All about the Dairy Group," ChooseMyPlate. gov, U.S. Department of Agriculture (USDA), July 29, 2016.

What Counts As A Cup In The Dairy Group?

In general, 1 cup of milk, yogurt or soymilk (soy beverage), 1 ½ ounces of natural cheese or 2 ounces of processed cheese can be considered as 1 cup from the Dairy Group.

Selection Tips

- Choose fat-free or low-fat milk, yogurt, and cheese. If you choose milk or yogurt that is not fat-free or cheese that is not low-fat, the fat in the product counts against your maximum limit for "empty calories" (calories from solid fats and added sugars).

- If sweetened milk products are chosen (flavored milk, yogurt, drinkable yogurt, desserts), the added sugars also count against your maximum limit for "empty calories".

- For those who are lactose intolerant, smaller portions (such as 4 fluid ounces of milk) may be well tolerated. Lactose-free and lower-lactose products are available. These include lactose-reduced or lactose-free milk, yogurt, and cheese, and calcium-fortified soymilk (soy beverage). Also, enzyme preparations can be added to milk to lower the lactose content.

- Calcium choices for those who do not consume dairy products include: kale leaves

- Calcium-fortified juices, cereals, breads, rice milk or almond milk. Calcium-fortified foods and beverages may not provide the other nutrients found in dairy products. Check the labels.

- Canned fish (sardines, salmon with bones) soybeans and other soy products (tofu made with calcium sulfate, soy yogurt, tempeh), some other beans, and some leafy greens (collard and turnip greens, kale, bok choy). The amount of calcium that can be absorbed from these foods varies.

Nutrients And Health Benefits

Consuming dairy products provides health benefits–especially improved bone health. Foods in the Dairy Group provide nutrients that are vital for health and maintenance of your body. These nutrients include calcium, potassium, vitamin D, and protein.

Nutrients

- Calcium is used for building bones and teeth and in maintaining bone mass. Dairy products are the primary source of calcium in American diets. Diets that provide 3 cups or the equivalent of dairy products per day can improve bone mass.

- Diets rich in potassium may help to maintain healthy blood pressure. Dairy products, especially yogurt, fluid milk, and soymilk (soy beverage), provide potassium.

- Vitamin D functions in the body to maintain proper levels of calcium and phosphorous, thereby helping to build and maintain bones. Milk and soymilk (soy beverage) that are fortified with vitamin D are good sources of this nutrient. Other sources include vitamin D-fortified yogurt and vitamin D-fortified ready-to-eat breakfast cereals.

- Milk products that are consumed in their low-fat or fat-free forms provide little or no solid fat.

Health Benefits

- Intake of dairy products is linked to improved bone health, and may reduce the risk of osteoporosis.

- The intake of dairy products is especially important to bone health during childhood and adolescence, when bone mass is being built.

- Intake of dairy products is also associated with a reduced risk of cardiovascular disease and type 2 diabetes, and with lower blood pressure in adults.

Why Is It Important To Make Fat-free Or Low-fat Choices From The Dairy Group?

Choosing foods from the Dairy Group that are high in saturated fats and cholesterol can have health implications. Diets high in saturated fats raise "bad" cholesterol levels in the blood. The "bad" cholesterol is called LDL (low-density lipoprotein) cholesterol. High LDL cholesterol, in turn, increases the risk for coronary heart disease. Many cheeses, whole milk, and products made from them are high in saturated fat. To help keep blood cholesterol levels healthy, limit the amount of these foods you eat. In addition, a high intake of fats makes it difficult to avoid consuming more calories than are needed.

Non-dairy Sources Of Calcium
For Those Who Choose Not To Consume Milk Products

Calcium choices for those who do not consume dairy products include:

- Calcium-fortified juices, cereals, breads, rice milk or almond milk.

- Canned fish (sardines, salmon with bones) soybeans and other soy products (tofu made with calcium sulfate, soy yogurt, tempeh), some other beans, and some leafy greens (collard and turnip greens, kale, bok choy). The amount of calcium that can be absorbed from these foods varies.

Tips For Taking Dairy Products

- Include milk or calcium-fortified soymilk (soy beverage) as a beverage at meals. Choose fat-free or low-fat milk.

- If you usually drink whole milk, switch gradually to fat-free milk, to lower saturated fat and calories. Try reduced fat (2%), then low-fat fruits and yogurt (1%), and finally fat-free (skim).

- If you drink cappuccinos or lattes—ask for them with fat-free (skim) milk.

- Add fat-free or low-fat milk instead of water to oatmeal and hot cereals.

- Use fat-free or low-fat milk when making condensed cream soups (such as cream of tomato).

- Have fat-free or low-fat yogurt as a snack.

- Make a dip for fruits or vegetables from yogurt.

- Make fruit-yogurt smoothies in the blender.

- For dessert, make chocolate or butterscotch pudding with fat-free or low-fat milk.

- Top cut-up fruit with flavored yogurt for a quick dessert.

- Top casseroles, soups, stews or vegetables with shredded reduced-fat or low-fat cheese.

- Top a baked potato with fat-free or low-fat yogurt.

Keep It Safe

- Avoid raw (unpasteurized) milk or any products made from unpasteurized milk.

- Chill (refrigerate) perishable food promptly and defrost foods properly. Refrigerate or freeze perishables, prepared food and leftovers as soon as possible. If food has been left at temperatures between 40° and 140° F for more than two hours, discard it, even though it may look and smell good.

- Separate raw, cooked, and ready-to-eat foods.

For Those Who Choose Not To Consume Milk Products

- If you avoid milk because of lactose intolerance, the most reliable way to get the health benefits of dairy products is to choose lactose-free alternatives within the Dairy Group, such as cheese, yogurt, lactose-free milk, or calcium-fortified soymilk (soy beverage)—or to consume the enzyme lactase before consuming milk.

- If you avoid milk for other reasons, choose non-dairy calcium choices such as:

  - Calcium-fortified juices, cereals, breads, rice milk, almond milk, or calcium-fortified soymilk (soy beverage).

  - Canned fish (sardines, salmon with bones) soybeans and other soy products (tofu made with calcium sulfate, soy yogurt, tempeh), some other beans, and some leafy greens (collard and turnip greens, kale, bok choy). The amount of calcium that can be absorbed from these foods varies.

Chapter 8
The Protein Group

What Foods Are In The Protein Foods Group?

All foods made from meat, poultry, seafood, beans and peas, eggs, processed soy products, nuts, and seeds are considered part of the Protein Foods Group. Beans and peas are also part of the Vegetable Group.

Select a variety of protein foods to improve nutrient intake and health benefits, including at least 8 ounces of cooked seafood per week. Young children need less, depending on their age and calorie needs. The advice to consume seafood does not apply to vegetarians. Vegetarian options in the Protein Foods Group include beans and peas, processed soy products, and nuts and seeds. Meat and poultry choices should be lean or low-fat.

How Much Food From The Protein Foods Group Is Daily?

The amount of food from the Protein Foods Group you need to eat depends on age, sex, and level of physical activity. Most Americans eat enough food from this group, but need to make leaner and more varied selections of these foods. Recommended daily amounts are shown in the table below.

About This Chapter: Information in this chapter is excerpted from "All about the Protein Foods Group," ChooseMyPlate.gov, U.S. Department of Agriculture (USDA), July 29, 2016.

Table 8.1. Daily Protein Foods Table

Daily Recommendation*

Girls	9–13 years old	5 ounce equivalents
	14–18 years old	5 ounce equivalents
Boys	9–13 years old	5 ounce equivalents
	14–18 years old	6 ½ ounce equivalents

These amounts are appropriate for individuals who get less than 30 minutes per day of moderate physical activity, beyond normal daily activities. Those who are more physically active may be able to consume more while staying within calorie needs.

What Counts As An Ounce-Equivalent In The Protein Foods Group?

In general, 1 ounce of meat, poultry or fish, ¼ cup cooked beans, 1 egg, 1 tablespoon of peanut butter or ½ ounce of nuts or seeds can be considered as 1 ounce-equivalent from the Protein Foods Group.

Selection Tips

- Choose lean or low-fat meat and poultry. If higher fat choices are made, such as regular ground beef (75–80% lean) or chicken with skin, the fat counts against your maximum limit for empty calories (calories from solid fats or added sugars).

- If solid fat is added in cooking, such as frying chicken in shortening or frying eggs in butter or stick margarine, this also counts against your maximum limit for empty calories.

- Select some seafood that is rich in omega-3 fatty acids, such as salmon, trout, sardines, anchovies, herring, Pacific oysters, and Atlantic and Pacific mackerel.

- Processed meats such as ham, sausage, frankfurters, and luncheon or deli meats have added sodium. Check the Nutrition Facts label to help limit sodium intake. Fresh chicken, turkey, and pork that have been enhanced with a salt-containing solution also have added sodium. Check the product label for statements such as "self-basting" or "contains up to__percent of__", which mean that a sodium-containing solution has been added to the product.

- Choose unsalted nuts and seeds to keep sodium intake low.

Why Is It Important To Make Lean Or Low-fat Choices From The Protein Foods Group?

Foods in the meat, poultry, fish, eggs, nuts, and seed group provide nutrients that are vital for health and maintenance of your body. However, choosing foods from this group that are high in saturated fat and cholesterol may have health implications.

The table below lists specific amounts that count as 1 ounce equivalent in the Protein Foods Group towards your daily recommended intake:

Table 8.2. Protein Foods Group Towards Your Daily Recommended Intake

	Amount That Counts As 1 Ounce Equivalent In The Protein Foods Group	**Common Portions And Ounce Equivalents**
Meats	1 ounce cooked lean beef 1 ounce cooked lean pork or ham	1 small steak (eye of round, filet) = 3/12 to 4 ounce equivalents 1 small lean hamburger = 2 to 3 ounce equivalents
Poultry	1 ounce cooked chicken or turkey, without skin 1 sandwich slice of turkey (4 1/2 x 2 1/2 x 1/8")	1 small chicken breast half = 3 ounce equivalents 1/2 Cornish game hen = 4 ounce equivalents
Seafood	1 ounce cooked fish or shell fish	1 can of tuna, drained = 3 to 4 ounce equivalents 1 salmon steak = 4 to 6 ounce equivalents 1 small trout = 3 ounce equivalents
Eggs	1 egg	3 egg whites = 2 ounce equivalents 3 egg yolks = 1 ounce equivalent
Beans and peas	1/2 ounce of nuts (12 almonds, 24 pistachios, 7 walnut halves) 1/2 ounce of seeds (pumpkin, sunflower or squash seeds, hulled, roasted) 1 Tablespoon of peanut butter or almond butter	1 ounce of nuts of seeds = 2 ounce equivalents

Table 8.2. Continued

	Amount That Counts As 1 Ounce Equivalent In The Protein Foods Group	Common Portions And Ounce Equivalents
Beans and peas	1/4 cup of cooked beans (such as black, kidney, pinto or white beans) 1/4 cup of cooked peas (such as chickpeas, cowpeas, lentils or split peas) 1/4 cup of baked beans, refried beans 1/4 cup (about 2 ounces) of tofu 1 ox. tempeh, cooked 1/4 cup roasted soybeans 1 falafel patty (2 1/4", 4 oz) 2 Tablespoons hummus	1 cup split pea soup = 2 ounce equivalents 1 cup lentil soup = 2 ounce equivalents 1 cup bean soup = 2 ounce equivalents 1 soy or bean burger patty = 2 ounce equivalents

Nutrients

- Diets that are high in saturated fats raise "bad" cholesterol levels in the blood. The "bad" cholesterol is called LDL (low-density lipoprotein) cholesterol. High LDL cholesterol, in turn, increases the risk for coronary heart disease. Some food choices in this group are high in saturated fat. These include fatty cuts of beef, pork, and lamb; regular (75% to 85% lean) ground beef; regular sausages, hot dogs, and bacon; some luncheon meats such as regular bologna and salami; and some poultry such as duck. To help keep blood cholesterol levels healthy, limit the amount of these foods you eat.

- Diets that are high in cholesterol can raise LDL cholesterol levels in the blood. Cholesterol is only found in foods from animal sources. Some foods from this group are high in cholesterol. These include egg yolks (egg whites are cholesterol-free) and organ meats such as liver and giblets. To help keep blood cholesterol levels healthy, limit the amount of these foods you eat.

- A high intake of fats makes it difficult to avoid consuming more calories than are needed.

Why Is It Important To Eat 8 Ounces Of Seafood Per Week?

- Seafood contains a range of nutrients, notably the omega-3 fatty acids, EPA, and DHA. Eating about 8 ounces per week of a variety of seafood contributes to the prevention of heart disease. Smaller amounts of seafood are recommended for young children.

- Seafood varieties that are commonly consumed in the United States that are higher in EPA and DHA and lower in mercury include salmon, anchovies, herring, sardines, Pacific oysters, trout, and Atlantic and Pacific mackerel (not king mackerel, which is high in mercury). The health benefits from consuming seafood outweigh the health risk associated with mercury, a heavy metal found in seafood in varying levels.

Health Benefits

- Meat, poultry, fish, dry beans and peas, eggs, nuts, and seeds supply many nutrients. These include protein, B vitamins (niacin, thiamin, riboflavin, and B6), vitamin E, iron, zinc, and magnesium.

- Proteins function as building blocks for bones, muscles, cartilage, skin, and blood. They are also building blocks for enzymes, hormones, and vitamins. Proteins are one of three nutrients that provide calories (the others are fat and carbohydrates).

- B vitamins found in this food group serve a variety of functions in the body. They help the body release energy, play a vital role in the function of the nervous system, aid in the formation of red blood cells, and help build tissues.

- Iron is used to carry oxygen in the blood. Many teenage girls have iron-deficiency anemia. They should eat foods high in heme iron (meats) or eat other non-heme iron containing foods along with a food rich in vitamin C, which can improve absorption of non-heme iron.

- Magnesium is used in building bones and in releasing energy from muscles.

- Zinc is necessary for biochemical reactions and helps the immune system function properly.

- EPA and DHA are omega-3 fatty acids found in varying amounts in seafood. Eating 8 ounces per week of seafood may help reduce the risk for heart disease.

What Are The Benefits Of Eating Nuts And Seeds?

Eating peanuts and certain tree nuts (i.e., walnuts, almonds, and pistachios) may reduce the risk of heart disease when consumed as part of a diet that is nutritionally adequate and within calorie needs. Because nuts and seeds are high in calories, eat them in small portions and use them to replace other protein foods, like some meat or poultry, rather than adding them to what you already eat. In addition, choose unsalted nuts and seeds to help reduce sodium intakes.

Vegetarian Choices In The Protein Foods Group

Vegetarians get enough protein from this group as long as the variety and amounts of foods selected are adequate. Protein sources from the Protein Foods Group for vegetarians include eggs (for ovo-vegetarians), beans and peas, nuts, nut butters, and soy products (tofu, tempeh, veggie burgers).

Tips To Help You Make Wise Choices From The Protein Foods Group

Go Lean With Protein

- The leanest beef cuts include round steaks and roasts (eye of round, top round, bottom round, round tip), top loin, top sirloin, and chuck shoulder and arm roasts.

- The leanest pork choices include pork loin, tenderloin, center loin, and ham.

- Choose lean ground beef. To be considered "lean," the product has to be at least 92% lean/8% fat.

- Buy skinless chicken parts, or take off the skin before cooking.

- Boneless skinless chicken breasts and turkey cutlets are the leanest poultry choices.

- Choose lean turkey, roast beef, ham, or low-fat luncheon meats for sandwiches instead of luncheon/deli meats with more fat, such as regular bologna or salami.

Vary Your Protein Choices

- Choose seafood at least twice a week as the main protein food. Look for seafood rich in omega-3 fatty acids, such as salmon, trout, and herring. Some ideas are:
  - Salmon steak or filet
  - Salmon loaf
  - Grilled or baked trout

- Choose beans, peas, or soy products as a main dish or part of a meal often. Some choices are:
  - Chili with kidney or pinto beans
  - Stir-fried tofu

- Split pea, lentil, minestrone, or white bean soups

- Baked beans

- Black bean enchiladas

- Garbanzo or kidney beans on a chef's salad

- Rice and beans

- Veggie burgers

- Hummus (chickpeas spread) on pita bread

- Choose unsalted nuts as a snack, on salads, or in main dishes. Use nuts to replace meat or poultry, *not in addition* to these items:

  - Use pine nuts in pesto sauce for pasta.

  - Add slivered almonds to steamed vegetables.

  - Add toasted peanuts or cashews to a vegetable stir fry instead of meat.

  - Sprinkle a few nuts on top of low-fat ice cream or frozen yogurt.

  - Add walnuts or pecans to a green salad instead of cheese or meat.

What To Look For On The Food Label

- Check the Nutrition Facts Label for the saturated fat, *trans*fat, cholesterol, and sodium content of packaged foods.

  - Processed meats such as hams, sausages, frankfurters, and luncheon or deli meats have added sodium. Check the ingredient and Nutrition Facts label to help limit sodium intake.

  - Fresh chicken, turkey, and pork that have been enhanced with a salt-containing solution also have added sodium. Check the product label for statements such as "self-basting" or "contains up to __% of __."

  - Lower fat versions of many processed meats are available. Look on the Nutrition Facts label to choose products with less fat and saturated fat.

Keep It Safe To Eat

- Separate raw, cooked and ready-to-eat foods.

- Do not wash or rinse meat or poultry.

- Wash cutting boards, knives, utensils and counter tops in hot soapy water after preparing each food item and before going on to the next one.

- Store raw meat, poultry and seafood on the bottom shelf of the refrigerator so juices don't drip onto other foods.

- Cook foods to a safe temperature to kill microorganisms. Use a meat thermometer, which measures the internal temperature of cooked meat and poultry, to make sure that the meat is cooked all the way through.

- Chill (refrigerate) perishable food promptly and defrost foods properly. Refrigerate or freeze perishables, prepared food and leftovers within two hours.

- Plan ahead to defrost foods. Never defrost food on the kitchen counter at room temperature. Thaw food by placing it in the refrigerator, submerging air-tight packaged food in cold tap water (change water every 30 minutes), or defrosting on a plate in the microwave.

- Avoid raw or partially cooked eggs or foods containing raw eggs and raw or undercooked meat and poultry.

- Women who may become pregnant, pregnant women, nursing mothers, and young children should avoid some types of fish and eat types lower in mercury. Call 1-888-SAFEFOOD (1-888-723-3366) for more information.

Chapter 9
Oils

What Are "Oils"?

Oils are fats that are liquid at room temperature, like the vegetable oils used in cooking. Oils come from many different plants and from fish. Oils are NOT a food group, but they provide essential nutrients. Therefore, oils are included in U.S. Department of Agriculture (USDA) food patterns.

Some **commonly eaten oils** include: canola oil, corn oil, cottonseed oil, olive oil, safflower oil, soybean oil, and sunflower oil. Some oils are used mainly as **flavorings**, such as walnut oil and sesame oil. A number of foods are naturally high in oils, like nuts, olives, some fish, and avocados.

Foods that are mainly oil include mayonnaise, certain salad dressings, and soft (tub or squeeze) margarine with no *trans* fats. Check the Nutrition Facts label to find margarines with 0 grams of *trans* fat. Amounts of *trans* fat are required to be listed on labels.

Most oils are high in monounsaturated or polyunsaturated fats, and low in saturated fats. Oils from plant sources (vegetable and nut oils) do not contain any cholesterol. In fact, no plant foods contain cholesterol. A few plant oils, however, including coconut oil, palm oil, and palm kernel oil, are high in saturated fats and for nutritional purposes should be considered to be solid fats.

About This Chapter: Information in this chapter is excerpted from "All about Oils," ChooseMyPlate.gov, U.S. Department of Agriculture (USDA), July 26, 2016.

Solid fats are fats that are solid at room temperature, like butter and shortening. Solid fats come from many animal foods and can be made from vegetable oils through a process called hydrogenation. Some common fats are: butter, milk fat, beef fat (tallow, suet), chicken fat, pork fat (lard), stick margarine, shortening, and partially hydrogenated oil.

How Much Is My Allowance For Oils?

Some Americans consume enough oil in the foods they eat, such as:

- nuts

- fish

- cooking oil

- salad dressing

Others could easily consume the recommended allowance by substituting oils for some solid fats they eat. A person's allowance for oils depends on age, sex, and level of physical activity. Daily allowances for oils are shown in the table below.

Table 9.1. Daily Allowance

Daily Allowance		
Girls	9–13 years old	5 teaspoons
	14–18 years old	5 teaspoons
Boys	9–13 years old	5 teaspoons
	14–18 years old	6 teaspoons

Why Is It Important To Consume Oils?

Most of the fats you eat should be polyunsaturated (PUFA) or monounsaturated (MUFA) fats. Oils are the major source of MUFAs and PUFAs in the diet. PUFAs contain some fatty acids that are necessary for health—called "essential fatty acids."

How Do I Count The Oils I Eat?

The table below gives a quick guide to the amount of oils in some common foods.

Table 9.2. Oil Table

Oils:	Amount of food	Amount of oil	Calories from oil	Total calories
		Teaspoons/grams	Approximate calories	Approximate calories
Vegetable oils (such as canola, corn, cottonseed, olive, peanut, safflower, soybean, and sunflower)	1 Tbsp	3 tsp/14 g	120	120
Foods rich in oils:				
Margarine, soft (*trans* fat free)	1 Tbsp	2 ½ tsp/11 g	100	100
Mayonnaise	1 Tbsp	2 ½ tsp/11 g	100	100
Mayonnaise-type salad dressing	1 Tbsp	1 tsp/5 g	45	55
Italian dressing	2 Tbsp	2 tsp/8 g	75	85
Thousand Island dressing	2 Tbsp	2 ½ tsp/11 g	100	120
Olives*, ripe, canned	4 large	½ tsp/ 2 g	15	20
Avocado*	½ med	3 tsp/15 g	130	160
Peanut butter*	2 T	4 tsp/16 g	140	190
Peanuts, dry roasted*	1 oz	3 tsp/14 g	120	165
Mixed nuts, dry roasted*	1 oz	3 tsp/14 g	130	170
Cashews, dry roasted*	1 oz	3 tsp/14 g	115	165
Almonds, dry roasted*	1 oz	3 tsp/14 g	130	170
Hazelnuts*	1 oz	4 tsp/ 18 g	160	185
Sunflower seeds*	1 oz	3 tsp/14 g	120	165

Avocados and olives are part of the Vegetable Group; nuts and seeds are part of the Protein Foods Group. These foods are also high in oils. Soft margarine, mayonnaise, and salad dressings are mainly oil and are not considered to be part of any food group.

Chapter 10
Empty Calories

Empty calories represented the sum of calories from solid fat and added sugars. Nearly 40 percent of total calories consumed (798 kcal/day of 2027 kcal) by 2–18 year olds were in the form of empty calories (433 kcal from solid fat and 365 kcal from added sugars, as shown in Table 10.1). This contrasts markedly with the discretionary calorie allowances, which range from 8 percent to 20 percent of total calories. As shown in Figure 10.1, consumption of empty calories far exceeded the corresponding discretionary calorie allowance for all sex-age groups.

Among 9–18 year olds, about half of these empty calories came from six specific foods: soda, fruit drinks, dairy desserts, grain desserts, pizza, and whole milk (Figure 10.1).

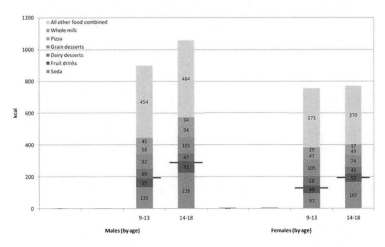

Figure 10.1. Consumption Of Empty Calories

About This Chapter: Information in this chapter is excerpted from "Dietary Sources of Energy, Solid Fats, and Added Sugars among Children and Adolescents in the United States," National Cancer Institute (NCI), May 2, 2016.

Table 10.1. Mean Intake And Major Sources Of Energy, Solid Fats And Added Sugars Among Adolescents In The United States (9–18 Years Old)

Top Sources

Age Group	#1	%	Mean (kcal)	SE	#2	%	Mean (kcal)	SE	#3	%	Mean (kcal)	SE	#4	%	Mean (kcal)	SE	#5	%	Mean (kcal)	SE
Energy																				
9–13	Grain desserts	7.1	145	15.6	Pizza	6.3	128	9.5	Chicken	6	122	13.1	Yeast breads	5.4	109	5.8	Soda	5.2	105	12.1
14–18	Soda	9.3	226	18.2	Pizza	8.8	213	24.5	Grain desserts	6.5	157	8.4	Yeast breads	6.2	151	14.5	Chicken	5.9	143	16.6
Solid Fats																				
9–13	Grain desserts	11.4	51	6	Pizza	11.2	50	5.2	Regular cheese	8.9	40	5.3	Whole milk	6.7	30	4.4	Fatty meats	6.5	29	2.9
14–18	Pizza	14.7	70	9.3	Grain desserts	9.7	46	2.8	Regular cheese	7.6	36	3.2	Fried potatoes	6.9	33	2.3	Fatty meats	5.7	27	3
Added Sugars																				
9–13	Soda	30.7	117	11.7	Fruit drinks	13.6	52	5.7	Grain desserts	12.4	47	5.6	Dairy desserts	8.8	33	5.2	Candy	7.8	30	3.1
14–18	Soda	44.5	197	9.7	Fruit drinks	14.1	63	5.6	Grain desserts	9.4	42	2.9	Candy	5.6	25	4.1	Dairy desserts	5.5	24	2.7

Solid fats and added sugars found in all other foods combined supplied the remainder. Sugar-sweetened beverages were the largest contributor, providing 22 percent of empty calories. In fact, among both males and females 9–13 and 14–18 years old, the empty calories consumed from soda and fruit drinks alone effectively "used up" or exceeded the discretionary calorie allowance.

Chapter 11
Water: Meeting Your Daily Fluid Needs

Water And Nutrition

Getting enough water every day is important for your health. Healthy people meet their fluid needs by drinking when thirsty and drinking with meals. Most of your fluid needs are met through the water and beverages you drink. However, you can get some fluids through the foods that you eat. For example, broth soups and foods with high water content such as celery, tomatoes or melons can contribute to fluid intake.

Water Helps Your Body

- Keep your temperature normal.
- Lubricate and cushion joints.
- Protect your spinal cord and other sensitive tissues.
- Get rid of wastes through urination, perspiration, and bowel movements.

Your Body Needs More Water When You Are:

- in hot climates
- more physically active

About This Chapter: Information in this chapter is from "Water and Nutrition," Centers for Disease Control and Prevention (CDC), June 3, 2014; information from "Community Water Fluoridation," Center for Disease Control and Prevention (CDC), April 7, 2015; information from "Make Better Beverage Choices," ChooseMyPlate.gov, U.S. Department of Agriculture (USDA), January 2016.

- running a fever

- having diarrhea or vomiting

If You Think You Are Not Getting Enough Water, These Tips May Help:

- Carry a water bottle for easy access when you are at work of running errands.

- Freeze some freezer safe water bottles. Take one with you for ice-cold water all day long.

- Choose water instead of sugar-sweetened beverages. This can also help with weight management. Substituting water for one 20-ounce sugar sweetened soda will save you about 240 calories. For example, during the school day students should have access to drinking water, giving them a healthy alternative to sugar-sweetened beverages.

- Choose water when eating out. Generally, you will save money and reduce calories.

- Add a wedge of lime or lemon to your water. This can help improve the taste and help you drink more water than you usually do.

Fluoride and Dental Health

The safety and benefits of fluoride are well documented. For 70 years, people in the United States have benefited from drinking water with fluoride, leading to better dental health.

Drinking fluoridated water keeps the teeth strong and reduced tooth decay by approximately 25 percent in children and adults.

Make Better Beverage Choices

What you drink is as important as what you eat. Many beverages contain added sugars and offer little or no nutrients, while others may provide nutrients but too much fat and too many calories. Here are some tips to help you make better beverage choices.

1. **Drink water**

   Drink water instead of sugary drinks. Regular soda, energy or sports drinks, and other sweet drinks usually contain a lot of added sugar, which provides more calories than needed.

2. How much water is enough?

Let your thirst be your guide. Water is an important nutrient for the body, but everyone's needs are different. Most of us get enough water from the foods we eat and the beverages we drink. A healthy body can balance water needs throughout the day. Drink plenty of water if you are very active, live or work in hot conditions, or are an older adult.

3. A thrifty option

Water is usually easy on the wallet. You can save money by drinking water from the tap at home or when eating out.

4. Manage your calories

Drink water with and between your meals. Adults and children take in about 400 calories per day as beverages—drinking water can help you manage your calories.

5. Kid-friendly drink zone

Make water, low-fat or fat-free milk, or 100% juice an easy option in your home. Have ready-to-go containers filled with water or healthy drinks available in the refrigerator. Place them in lunch boxes or backpacks for easy access when kids are away from home. Depending on age, children can drink ½ to 1 cup, and adults can drink up to 1 cup of 100% fruit or vegetable juice* each day.

6. Don't forget your dairy**

When you choose milk or milk alternatives, select low-fat or fat-free milk or fortified soymilk. Each type of milk offers the same key nutrients such as calcium, vitamin D, and potassium, but the number of calories are very different. Older children, teens, and adults need 3 cups of milk per day, while children 4 to 8 years old need 2½ cups and children 2 to 3 years old need 2 cups.

* 100% juice is part of the Fruit or Vegetable Group. Juice should make up half or less of total recommended fruit or vegetable intake.

** Milk is a part of the Dairy Group. A cup = 1 cup of milk or yogurt, 1½ ounces of natural cheese, or 2 ounces of processed cheese.

7. Enjoy your beverage

When water just won't do—enjoy the beverage of your choice, but just cut back. Remember to check the serving size and the number of servings in the can, bottle, or container to stay within calorie needs. Select smaller cans, cups, or glasses instead of large or super-sized options.

8. **Water on the go**

   Water is always convenient. Fill a clean, reusable water bottle and toss it in your bag or briefcase to quench your thirst throughout the day. Reusable bottles are also easy on the environment.

9. **Check the facts**

   Use the Nutrition Facts label to choose beverages at the grocery store. The food label and ingredients list contain information about added sugars, saturated fat, sodium, and calories to help you make better choices.

10. **Compare what you drink**

    Food-A-Pedia, an online feature available on the SuperTracker website (www.super-tracker.usda.gov/foodapedia.aspx), can help you compare calories, added sugars, and fats in your favorite beverages.

Part Two
Vitamins And Minerals

Chapter 12
Vitamin A And Carotenoids

What Is Vitamin A And What Does It Do?

Vitamin A is a fat-soluble vitamin that is naturally present in many foods. Vitamin A is important for normal vision, the immune system, and reproduction. Vitamin A also helps the heart, lungs, kidneys, and other organs work properly.

There are two different types of vitamin A. The first type, preformed vitamin A, is found in meat, poultry, fish, and dairy products. The second type, provitamin A, is found in fruits, vegetables, and other plant-based products. The most common type of provitamin A in foods and dietary supplements is beta-carotene.

How Much Vitamin A Do I Need?

The amount of vitamin A you need depends on your age and reproductive status. Recommended intakes for vitamin A for people aged 14 years and older range between 700 and 900 micrograms (mcg) of retinol activity equivalents (RAE) per day. Recommended intakes for women who are nursing range between 1,200 and 1,300 RAE. Lower values are recommended for infants and children younger than 14.

However, the vitamin A content of foods and dietary supplements is given on product labels in international units (IU), not mcg RAE. Converting between IU and mcg RAE is not easy. A varied diet with 900 mcg RAE of vitamin A, for example, provides between 3,000 and 36,000 IU of vitamin A depending on the foods consumed.

About This Chapter: Information in this chapter is excerpted from "Vitamin A," Office on Dietary Supplements (ODS), National Institutes of Health (NIH), June 5, 2013.

For adults and children aged 4 years and older, the U.S. Food and Drug Administration (FDA) has established a vitamin A Daily Value (DV) of 5,000 IU from a varied diet of both plant and animal foods. DVs are not recommended intakes; they don't vary by age and sex, for example. But trying to reach 100 percent of the DV each day, on average, is useful to help you get enough vitamin A.

What Foods Provide Vitamin A?

Vitamin A is found naturally in many foods and is added to some foods, such as milk and cereal. You can get recommended amounts of vitamin A by eating a variety of foods, including the following:

- Beef liver and other organ meats (but these foods are also high in cholesterol, so limit the amount you eat).
- Some types of fish, such as salmon.
- Green leafy vegetables and other green, orange, and yellow vegetables, such as broccoli, carrots, and squash.
- Fruits, including cantaloupe, apricots, and mangos.
- Dairy products, which are among the major sources of vitamin A for Americans.
- Fortified breakfast cereals.

What Kinds Of Vitamin A Dietary Supplements Are Available?

Vitamin A is available in dietary supplements, usually in the form of retinyl acetate or retinyl palmitate (preformed vitamin A), beta-carotene (provitamin A) or a combination of preformed and provitamin A. Most multivitamin-mineral supplements contain vitamin A. Dietary supplements that contain only vitamin A are also available.

Am I Getting Enough Vitamin A?

Most people in the United States get enough vitamin A from the foods they eat, and vitamin A deficiency is rare. However, certain groups of people are more likely than others to have trouble getting enough vitamin A:

- premature infants, who often have low levels of vitamin A in their first year
- infants, young children, pregnant women, and breastfeeding women in developing countries; and
- people with cystic fibrosis

What Are Some Effects Of Vitamin A On Health?

Scientists are studying vitamin A to understand how it affects health. Here are some examples of what this research has shown.

Cancer

People who eat a lot of foods containing beta-carotene might have a lower risk of certain kinds of cancer, such as lung cancer or prostate cancer. But studies to date have not shown that vitamin A or beta-carotene supplements can help prevent cancer or lower the chances of dying from this disease. In fact, studies show that smokers who take high doses of beta-carotene supplements have an increased risk of lung cancer.

Age-Related Macular Degeneration

Age-related macular degeneration (AMD) or the loss of central vision as people age, is one of the most common causes of vision loss in older people. Among people with AMD who are at high risk of developing advanced AMD, a supplement containing antioxidants, zinc, and copper with or without beta-carotene has shown promise for slowing down the rate of vision loss.

Measles

When children with vitamin A deficiency (which is rare in North America) get measles, the disease tends to be more severe. In these children, taking supplements with high doses of vitamin A can shorten the fever and diarrhea caused by measles. These supplements can also lower the risk of death in children with measles who live in developing countries where vitamin A deficiency is common.

Can Vitamin A Be Harmful?

Yes, high intakes of some forms of vitamin A can be harmful.

Getting too much preformed vitamin A (usually from supplements or certain medicines) can cause dizziness, nausea, headaches, coma, and even death. High intakes of preformed vitamin A in pregnant women can also cause birth defects in their babies. Women who might be pregnant should not take high doses of vitamin A supplements.

Consuming high amounts of beta-carotene or other forms of provitamin A can turn the skin yellow-orange, but this condition is harmless. High intakes of beta-carotene do not cause birth defects or the other more serious effects caused by getting too much preformed vitamin A.

The upper limit for preformed vitamin A in IU is listed below. This level does not apply to people who are taking vitamin A for medical reasons under the care of a doctor. Upper limits for beta-carotene and other forms of provitamin A have not been established.

Table 12.1. Upper Limit For Preformed Vitamin A In International Units (IU)

Life Stage	Upper Limit
Teens 14–18 years	9,333 IU

Chapter 13

B Vitamins

Folate

What Is Folate And What Does It Do?

Folate is a B-vitamin that is naturally present in many foods. A form of folate, called folic acid, is used in dietary supplements and fortified foods.

Our bodies need folate to make DNA and other genetic material. Folate is also needed for the body's cells to divide.

How Much Folate Do I Need?

The amount of folate you need depends on your age. Average daily recommended amounts is listed below in micrograms (mcg) of dietary folate equivalents (DFEs).

All women and teen girls who could become pregnant should consume 400 mcg of folic acid daily from supplements, fortified foods, or both in addition to the folate they get naturally from foods.

About This Chapter: Information in this chapter is excerpted from "Folate," Office of Dietary Supplements (ODS), National Institutes of Health (NIH) April 20, 2016; information from "Riboflavin," Office of Dietary Supplements (ODS), National Institutes of Health (NIH), February 17, 2016; information from "Thiamin," Office of Dietary Supplements (ODS), National Institutes of Health (NIH), April 13, 2016; information from "Vitamin B6," Office of Dietary Supplements (ODS), National Institutes of Health (NIH), February 17, 2016; and information from "Vitamin B12 Fact Sheet for Consumers," Office of Dietary Supplements (ODS), National Institutes of Health (NIH), February 17, 2016.

Table 13.1. Life Stages With Recommended Amount

Life Stage	Recommended Amount
Teens 14–18 years	400 mcg DFE

What Foods Provide Folate?

Folate is naturally present in many foods and food companies add folic acid to other foods, including bread, cereal, and pasta. You can get recommended amounts by eating a variety of foods, including the following:

- Vegetables (especially asparagus, Brussels sprouts, and dark green leafy vegetables such as spinach and mustard greens).
- Fruits and fruit juices (especially oranges and orange juice).
- Nuts, beans, and peas (such as peanuts, black-eyed peas, and kidney beans).
- Grains (including whole grains; fortified cold cereals; enriched flour products such as bread, bagels, cornmeal, and pasta; and rice).
- Folic acid is added to many grain-based products and corn masa flour (used to make corn tortillas and tamales, for example). To find out whether folic acid has been added to a food, check the product label.

Beef liver is high in folate but is also high in cholesterol, so limit the amount you eat. Only small amounts of folate are found in other animal foods like meats, poultry, seafood, eggs, and dairy products.

What Kinds Of Folic Acid Dietary Supplements Are Available?

Folic acid is available in multivitamins and prenatal vitamins. It is also available in B-complex dietary supplements and supplements containing only folic acid.

Am I Getting Enough Folate?

Most people in the United States get enough folate. However, certain groups of people are more likely than others to have trouble getting enough folate:

- Teen girls and women aged 14–30 years (especially before and during pregnancy).
- Non-Hispanic black women.
- People with disorders that lower nutrient absorption (such as celiac disease and inflammatory bowel disease).
- People with alcoholism.

What Happens If I Don't Get Enough Folate?

Folate deficiency is rare in the United States, but some people get barely enough. Getting too little folate can result in megaloblastic anemia, which causes weakness, fatigue, trouble concentrating, irritability, headache, heart palpitations, and shortness of breath. Folate deficiency can also cause open sores on the tongue and inside the mouth as well as changes in the color of the skin, hair, or fingernails.

Women who don't get enough folate are at risk of having babies with neural tube defects, such as spina bifida. Folate deficiency can also increase the likelihood of having a premature or low-birth-weight baby.

What Are Some Effects Of Folate On Health?

Scientists are studying folate to understand how it affects health. Here are several examples of what this research has shown.

Neural Tube Defects

Taking folic acid regularly before becoming pregnant and during early pregnancy helps prevent neural tube defects in babies. But about half of all pregnancies are unplanned. Therefore, all women and teen girls who could become pregnant should consume 400 mcg of folic acid daily from supplements, fortified foods, or both in addition to the folate they get naturally from foods.

Since 1998, the U.S. Food and Drug Administration (FDA) has required food companies to add folic acid to enriched bread, cereal, flour, cornmeal, pasta, rice, and other grain products sold in the United States. Because most people in the United States eat these foods on a regular basis, folic acid intakes have increased and the number of babies born with neural tube defects has decreased since 1998.

Preterm Birth, Congenital Heart Defects, And Other Birth Defects

Taking folic acid might reduce the risk of having a premature baby and prevent birth defects, such as congenital heart problems. But more research is needed to understand how folic acid affects the risk of these conditions.

Cancer

Folate that is found naturally in food may decrease the risk of several forms of cancer. But folate might have different effects depending on how much is taken and when. Modest amounts of folic acid taken before cancer develops might decrease cancer risk, but high doses taken after cancer (especially colorectal cancer) begins might speed up its progression. For this reason, high doses of folic acid supplements (more than the upper limit of 1,000 mcg) should be taken with caution, especially by people who have a history of colorectal adenomas (which sometimes turn into cancer). More research is needed to understand the roles of dietary folate and folic acid supplements in cancer risk.

Heart Disease And Stroke

Some scientists used to think that folic acid and other B-vitamins might reduce heart disease risk by lowering levels of homocysteine, an amino acid in the blood. But although folic acid supplements do lower blood homocysteine levels, they don't decrease the risk of heart disease. Some studies have shown that a combination of folic acid with other B-vitamins, however, helps prevent stroke.

Depression

People with low blood levels of folate might be more likely to suffer from depression and might not respond as well to treatment with antidepressants as people with normal folate levels.

Folic acid supplements might make antidepressant medications more effective. But it is not clear whether these supplements help people with both normal folate levels and those with folate deficiency. More research is needed to learn about the role of folate in depression and whether folic acid supplements are helpful when used in combination with standard treatment.

Can Folate Be Harmful?

Folate that is naturally present in food is not harmful. Folic acid in supplements and forti-fied foods, however, should not be consumed in amounts above the upper limit, unless recom-mended by a healthcare provider.

Taking large amounts of folic acid might hide a vitamin B12 deficiency. Folic acid can cor-rect the anemia but not the nerve damage caused by vitamin B12 deficiency. This can lead to permanent damage of the brain, spinal cord, and nerves. High doses of folic acid might also increase the risk of colorectal cancer and possibly other cancers in some people.

The upper limit for folic acid is listed below.

Table 13.2. Upper Limit For Folic Acid

Ages	Upper Limit
Teens 14–18 years	800 mcg

Riboflavin

What Is Riboflavin And What Does It Do?

Riboflavin (also called vitamin B2) is important for the growth, development, and function of the cells in your body. It also helps turn the food you eat into the energy you need.

How Much Riboflavin Do I Need?

The amount of riboflavin you need depends on your age and sex. Average daily recommended amounts are listed below in milligrams (mg).

Table 13.3. Average Daily Recommended Amount Of Riboflavin

Life Stage	Recommended Amount
Teen boys 14–18 years	1.3 mg
Teen girls 14–18 years	1 mg

What Foods Provide Riboflavin?

Riboflavin is found naturally in some foods and is added to many fortified foods. You can get recommended amounts of riboflavin by eating a variety of foods, including the following:

- eggs, organ meats (such as kidneys and liver), lean meats, and low-fat milk
- green vegetables (such as asparagus, broccoli, and spinach)
- fortified cereals, bread, and grain products

What Kinds Of Riboflavin Dietary Supplements Are Available?

Riboflavin is found in multivitamin/multimineral supplements, in B-complex dietary supplements, and in supplements containing only riboflavin. Some supplements have much more than the recommended amounts of riboflavin, but your body can't absorb more than about 27 mg at a time.

What Is An Effect Of Riboflavin Supplements On Health?

Scientists are studying riboflavin to better understand how it affects health. Here is an example of what this research has shown.

Migraine Headache

Some studies show that riboflavin supplements might help prevent migraine headaches, but other studies do not. Riboflavin supplements usually have very few side effects, so some medical experts recommend trying riboflavin, under the guidance of a healthcare provider, for preventing migraines.

Can Riboflavin Be Harmful?

Riboflavin has not been shown to cause any harm.

Thiamin

What Is Thiamin And What Does It Do?

Thiamin (also called vitamin B1) helps turn the food you eat into the energy you need. Thiamin is important for the growth, development, and function of the cells in your body.

How Much Thiamin Do I Need?

The amount of thiamin you need depends on your age and sex. Average daily recommended amounts are listed below in milligrams (mg).

Table 13.4. Average Daily Recommended Amount Of Thiamin

Life Stage	Recommended Amount
Teen boys 14–18 years	1.2 mg
Teen girls 14–18 years	1 mg

What Foods Provide Thiamin?

Thiamin is found naturally in many foods and is added to some fortified foods. You can get recommended amounts of thiamin by eating a variety of foods, including the following:

- whole grains and fortified bread, cereal, pasta, and rice
- meat (especially pork) and fish
- legumes (such as black beans and soybeans), seeds, and nuts

What Kinds Of Thiamin Dietary Supplements Are Available?

Thiamin is found in multivitamin/multimineral supplements, in B-complex dietary supplements, and in supplements containing only thiamin. Common forms of thiamin in dietary supplements are thiamin mononitrate and thiamin hydrochloride. Some supplements use a synthetic form of thiamin called benfotiamine.

What Are Some Effects Of Thiamin On Health?

Scientists are studying thiamin to better understand how it affects health. Here are some examples of what this research has shown.

Diabetes

People with diabetes often have low levels of thiamin in their blood. Scientists are studying whether thiamin supplements can improve blood sugar levels and glucose tolerance in people with type 2 diabetes. They are also studying whether benfotiamine (a synthetic form of thiamin) supplements can help with nerve damage caused by diabetes.

Heart Failure

Many people with heart failure have low levels of thiamin. Scientists are studying whether thiamin supplements might help people with heart failure.

Can Thiamin Be Harmful?

Thiamin has not been shown to cause any harm.

What Happens If I Don't Get Enough Vitamin A?

Vitamin A deficiency is rare in the United States, although it is common in many developing countries. The most common symptom of vitamin A deficiency in young children and pregnant women is an eye condition called xerophthalmia. Xerophthalmia is the inability to see in low light, and it can lead to blindness if it isn't treated.

Vitamin B6

What Is Vitamin B6 And What Does It Do?

Vitamin B6 is a vitamin that is naturally present in many foods. The body needs vitamin B6 for more than 100 enzyme reactions involved in metabolism. Vitamin B6 is also involved in brain development during pregnancy and infancy as well as immune function.

How Much Vitamin B6 Do I Need?

The amount of vitamin B6 you need depends on your age. Average daily recommended amounts are listed below in milligrams (mg).

Table 13.5. Average Daily Recommended Amount Of Vitamin B6

Life Stage	Recommended Amount
Teens 14–18 years (boys)	1.3 mg
Teens 14–18 years (girls)	1.2 mg

What Foods Provide Vitamin B6?

Vitamin B6 is found naturally in many foods and is added to other foods. You can get recommended amounts of vitamin B6 by eating a variety of foods, including the following:

- poultry, fish, and organ meats, all rich in vitamin B6
- potatoes and other starchy vegetables, which are some of the major sources of vitamin B6 for Americans
- fruit (other than citrus), which are also among the major sources of vitamin B6 for Americans

What Kinds Of Vitamin B6 Dietary Supplements Are Available?

Vitamin B6 is available in dietary supplements, usually in the form of pyridoxine. Most multivitamin-mineral supplements contain vitamin B6. Dietary supplements that contain only vitamin B6 or vitamin B6 with other B vitamins, are also available.

What Are Some Effects Of Vitamin B6 On Health?

Scientists are studying vitamin B6 to understand how it affects health. Here are some examples of what this research has shown.

Heart Disease

Some scientists had thought that certain B vitamins (such as folic acid, vitamin B12, and vitamin B6) might reduce heart disease risk by lowering levels of homocysteine, an amino acid in the blood. Although vitamin B supplements do lower blood homocysteine, research shows that they do not actually reduce the risk or severity of heart disease or stroke.

Cancer

People with low levels of vitamin B6 in the blood might have a higher risk of certain kinds of cancer, such as colorectal cancer. But studies to date have not shown that vitamin B6 supplements can help prevent cancer or lower the chances of dying from this disease.

Cognitive Function

Some research indicates that elderly people who have higher blood levels of vitamin B6 have better memory. However, taking vitamin B6 supplements (alone or combined with vitamin B12 and/or folic acid) does not seem to improve cognitive function or mood in healthy people or in people with dementia.

Premenstrual Syndrome

Scientists aren't yet certain about the potential benefits of taking vitamin B6 for premenstrual syndrome (PMS). But some studies show that vitamin B6 supplements could reduce PMS symptoms, including moodiness, irritability, forgetfulness, bloating, and anxiety.

Nausea And Vomiting In Pregnancy

At least half of all women experience nausea, vomiting or both in the first few months of pregnancy. Based on the results of several studies, the American Congress of Obstetricians and Gynecologists (ACOG) recommends taking vitamin B6 supplements under a doctor's care for nausea and vomiting during pregnancy.

Can Vitamin B6 Be Harmful?

People almost never get too much vitamin B6 from food. But taking high levels of vitamin B6 from supplements for a year or longer can cause severe nerve damage, leading people to lose control of their bodily movements. The symptoms usually stop when they stop taking the supplements. Other symptoms of too much vitamin B6 include painful, unsightly skin patches, extreme sensitivity to sunlight, nausea, and heartburn.

The upper limit for vitamin B6 is listed below. This level does not apply to people who are taking vitamin B6 for medical reasons under the care of a doctor.

Table 13.6. Upper Limit For Vitamin B6

Life Stage	Upper Limit
Teens 14–18 years	80 mg

Vitamin B12

What Is Vitamin B12 And What Does It Do?

Vitamin B12 is a nutrient that helps keep the body's nerve and blood cells healthy and helps make DNA, the genetic material in all cells. Vitamin B12 also helps prevent a type of anemia called megaloblastic anemia that makes people tired and weak.

Two steps are required for the body to absorb vitamin B12 from food. First, hydrochloric acid in the stomach separates vitamin B12 from the protein to which vitamin B12 is attached in food. After this, vitamin B12 combines with a protein made by the stomach called intrinsic factor and is absorbed by the body. Some people have pernicious anemia, a condition where they cannot make intrinsic factor. As a result, they have trouble absorbing vitamin B12 from all foods and dietary supplements.

How Much Vitamin B12 Do I Need?

The amount of vitamin B12 you need each day depends on your age. Average daily recommended amounts for different ages are listed below in micrograms (mcg):

Table 13.7. Average Daily Recommended Amount Of Vitamin B12

Life Stage	Recommended Amount
Teens 14–18 years (boys)	1.3 mg
Teens 14–18 years (girls)	1.2 mg

What Foods Provide Vitamin B12?

Vitamin B12 is found naturally in a wide variety of animal foods and is added to some fortified foods. Plant foods have no vitamin B12 unless they are fortified. You can get recommended amounts of vitamin B12 by eating a variety of foods including the following:

- Beef liver and clams, which are the best sources of vitamin B12.
- Fish, meat, poultry, eggs, milk, and other dairy products, which also contain vitamin B12.
- Some breakfast cereals, nutritional yeasts, and other food products that are fortified with vitamin B12. To find out if vitamin B12 has been added to a food product, check the product labels.

What Kinds Of Vitamin B12 Dietary Supplements Are Available?

Vitamin B12 is found in almost all multivitamins. Dietary supplements that contain only vitamin B12 or vitamin B12 with nutrients such as folic acid and other B vitamins, are also available. Check the Supplement Facts label to determine the amount of vitamin B12 provided.

Vitamin B12 is also available in sublingual forms (which are dissolved under the tongue). There is no evidence that sublingual forms are better absorbed than pills that are swallowed.

A prescription form of vitamin B12 can be administered as a shot. This is usually used to treat vitamin B12 deficiency. Vitamin B12 is also available as a prescription medication in nasal gel form (for use in the nose).

What Are Some Effects Of Vitamin B12 On Health?

Scientists are studying vitamin B12 to see how it affects health. Here are several examples of what this research has shown.

Heart Disease

Vitamin B12 supplements (along with folic acid and vitamin B6) do not reduce the risk of getting heart disease. Scientists had thought that these vitamins might be helpful because they reduce blood levels of homocysteine, a compound linked to an increased risk of having a heart attack or stroke. Vitamin B12 supplements (along with folic acid and vitamin B6) do not reduce the risk of getting heart disease. Scientists had thought that these vitamins might be helpful because they reduce blood levels of homocysteine, a compound linked to an increased risk of having a heart attack or stroke.

Energy And Athletic Performance

Advertisements often promote vitamin B12 supplements as a way to increase energy or endurance. Except in people with a vitamin B12 deficiency, no evidence shows that vitamin B12 supplements increase energy or improve athletic performance.

Can Vitamin B12 Be Harmful?

Vitamin B12 has not been shown to cause any harm.

Chapter 14
Vitamin C

What Is Vitamin C And What Does It Do?

Vitamin C, also known as ascorbic acid, is a water-soluble nutrient found in some foods. In the body, it acts as an antioxidant, helping to protect cells from the damage caused by free radicals. Free radicals are compounds formed when our bodies convert the food we eat into energy. People are also exposed to free radicals in the environment from cigarette smoke, air pollution, and ultraviolet light from the sun.

The body also needs vitamin C to make collagen, a protein required to help wounds heal. In addition, vitamin C improves the absorption of iron from plant-based foods and helps the immune system work properly to protect the body from disease.

How Much Vitamin C Do I Need?

The amount of vitamin C you need each day depends on your age. Average daily recommended amounts for different ages are listed below in milligrams (mg).

Table 14.1. Average Daily Recommended Amounts Of Vitamin C

Life Stage	Recommended Amount
Teens 14–18 years (boys)	75 mg
Teens 14–18 years (girls)	65 mg

If you smoke, add 35 mg to the above values to calculate your total daily recommended amount.

About This Chapter: Information in this chapter is excerpted from "Vitamin C," Office on Dietary Supplements (ODS), National Institutes of Health (NIH), June 24, 2011. Reviewed September 2016.

What Foods Provide Vitamin C?

Fruits and vegetables are the best sources of vitamin C. You can get recommended amounts of vitamin C by eating a variety of foods including the following:

- Citrus fruits (such as oranges and grapefruit) and their juices, as well as red and green pepper and kiwifruit, which have a lot of vitamin C.
- Other fruits and vegetables—such as broccoli, strawberries, cantaloupe, baked potatoes, and tomatoes—which also have vitamin C.
- Some foods and beverages that are fortified with vitamin C. To find out if vitamin C has been added to a food product, check the product labels.

The vitamin C content of food may be reduced by prolonged storage and by cooking. Steaming or microwaving may lessen cooking losses. Fortunately, many of the best food sources of vitamin C, such as fruits and vegetables, are usually eaten raw.

What Kinds Of Vitamin C Dietary Supplements Are Available?

Most multivitamins have vitamin C. Vitamin C is also available alone as a dietary supplement or in combination with other nutrients. The vitamin C in dietary supplements is usually in the form of ascorbic acid, but some supplements have other forms, such as sodium ascorbate, calcium ascorbate, other mineral ascorbates, and ascorbic acid with bioflavonoids. Research has not shown that any form of vitamin C is better than the other forms.

What Are Some Effects Of Vitamin C On Health?

Scientists are studying vitamin C to understand how it affects health. Here are several examples of what this research has shown.

Cancer Prevention And Treatment

People with high intakes of vitamin C from fruits and vegetables might have a lower risk of getting many types of cancer, such as lung, breast, and colon cancer. However, taking vitamin C supplements, with or without other antioxidants, doesn't seem to protect people from getting cancer.

It is not clear whether taking high doses of vitamin C is helpful as a treatment for cancer. Vitamin C's effects appear to depend on how it is administered to the patient. Oral doses of vitamin C can't raise blood levels of vitamin C nearly as high as intravenous doses given through injections. A few studies in animals and test tubes indicate that very high blood levels of vitamin C might shrink tumors. But more research is needed to determine whether high-dose intravenous vitamin C helps treat cancer in people.

Vitamin C dietary supplements and other antioxidants might interact with chemotherapy and radiation therapy for cancer. People being treated for cancer should talk with their oncologist before taking vitamin C or other antioxidant supplements, especially in high doses.

Cardiovascular Disease

People who eat lots of fruits and vegetables seem to have a lower risk of cardiovascular disease. Researchers believe that the antioxidant content of these foods might be partly responsible for this association because oxidative damage is a major cause of cardiovascular disease. However, scientists aren't sure whether vitamin C itself, either from food or supplements, helps protect people from cardiovascular disease. It is also not clear whether vitamin C helps prevent cardiovascular disease from getting worse in people who already have it.

Age-Related Macular Degeneration (AMD) And Cataracts

AMD and cataracts are two of the leading causes of vision loss in older people. Researchers do not believe that vitamin C and other antioxidants affect the risk of getting AMD. However, research suggests that vitamin C combined with other nutrients might help slow AMD progression.

In a large study among older people with AMD who were at high risk of developing advanced AMD, those who took a daily dietary supplement with 500 mg vitamin C, 80 mg zinc, 400 IU vitamin E, 15 mg beta-carotene, and 2 mg copper for about 6 years had a lower chance of developing advanced AMD. They also had less vision loss than those who did not take the dietary supplement. People who have or are developing the disease might want to talk with their doctor about taking dietary supplements.

The relationship between vitamin C and cataract formation is unclear. Some studies show that people who get more vitamin C from foods have a lower risk of getting cataracts. But further research is needed to clarify this association and to determine whether vitamin C supplements affect the risk of getting cataracts.

The Common Cold Myth

Although vitamin C has long been a popular remedy for the common cold, research shows that for most people, vitamin C supplements do not reduce the risk of getting the common cold. However, people who take vitamin C supplements regularly might have slightly shorter colds or somewhat milder symptoms when they do have a cold. Using vitamin C supplements after cold symptoms start does not appear to be helpful.

Can Vitamin C Be Harmful?

Taking too much vitamin C can cause diarrhea, nausea, and stomach cramps. In people with a condition called hemochromatosis, which causes the body to store too much iron, high doses of vitamin C could worsen iron overload and damage body tissues.

The upper limit for vitamin C is listed below:

Table 14.2. Upper Limit For Vitamin C

Life Stage	Upper Limit
Teens 14–18 years	1,800 mg

Chapter 15
Vitamin D

What Is Vitamin D And What Does It Do?

Vitamin D is a nutrient found in some foods that is needed for health and to maintain strong bones. It does so by helping the body absorb calcium (one of bone's main building blocks) from food and supplements. People who get too little vitamin D may develop soft, thin, and brittle bones, a condition known as rickets in children and osteomalacia in adults.

Vitamin D is important to the body in many other ways as well. Muscles need it to move, for example, nerves need it to carry messages between the brain and every body part, and the immune system needs vitamin D to fight off invading bacteria and viruses. Together with calcium, vitamin D also helps protect older adults from osteoporosis. Vitamin D is found in cells throughout the body.

How Much Vitamin D Do I Need?

The amount of vitamin D you need each day depends on your age. Average daily recommended amount from the Food and Nutrition Board (a national group of experts) for different ages is listed below in International Units (IU):

Table 15.1. Average Daily Recommended Amount Of Vitamin D

Life Stage	Recommended Amount
Teens 14–18 years	600 IU

About This Chapter: Information in this chapter is excerpted from "Vitamin D Fact Sheet for Consumers," Office on Dietary Supplements (ODS), National Institutes of Health (NIH), April 15, 2016.

What Foods Provide Vitamin D?

Very few foods naturally have vitamin D. Fortified foods provide most of the vitamin D in American diets.

- Fatty fish such as salmon, tuna, and mackerel are among the best sources.
- Beef liver, cheese, and egg yolks provide small amounts.
- Mushrooms provide some vitamin D. In some mushrooms that are newly available in stores, the vitamin D content is being boosted by exposing these mushrooms to ultraviolet light.
- Almost all of the U.S. milk supply is fortified with 400 IU of vitamin D per quart. But foods made from milk, like cheese and ice cream, are usually not fortified.
- Vitamin D is added to many breakfast cereals and to some brands of orange juice, yogurt, margarine, and soy beverages; check the labels.

Can I Get Vitamin D From The Sun?

The body makes vitamin D when skin is directly exposed to the sun, and most people meet at least some of their vitamin D needs this way. Skin exposed to sunshine indoors through a window will not produce vitamin D. Cloudy days, shade, and having dark-colored skin also cut down on the amount of vitamin D the skin makes.

However, despite the importance of the sun to vitamin D synthesis, it is prudent to limit exposure of skin to sunlight in order to lower the risk for skin cancer. When out in the sun for more than a few minutes, wear protective clothing and apply sunscreen with an SPF (sun protection factor) of 8 or more. Tanning beds also cause the skin to make vitamin D, but pose similar risks for skin cancer.

People who avoid the sun or who cover their bodies with sunscreen or clothing should include good sources of vitamin D in their diets or take a supplement. Recommended intakes of vitamin D are set on the assumption of little sun exposure.

What Kinds Of Vitamin D Dietary Supplements Are Available?

Vitamin D is found in supplements (and fortified foods) in two different forms: D2 (ergocalciferol) and D3 (cholecalciferol). Both increase vitamin D in the blood.

What Are Some Effects Of Vitamin D On Health?

Vitamin D is being studied for its possible connections to several diseases and medical problems, including diabetes, hypertension, and autoimmune conditions such as multiple sclerosis. Two of them discussed below are bone disorders and some types of cancer.

Bone Disorders

As they get older, millions of people (mostly women, but men too) develop, or are at risk of, osteoporosis, where bones become fragile and may fracture if one falls. It is one consequence of not getting enough calcium and vitamin D over the long term. Supplements of both vitamin D3 (at 700–800 IU/day) and calcium (500–1,200 mg/day) have been shown to reduce the risk of bone loss and fractures.

Cancer

Some studies suggest that vitamin D may protect against colon cancer and perhaps even cancers of the prostate and breast. But higher levels of vitamin D in the blood have also been linked to higher rates of pancreatic cancer. At this time, it's too early to say whether low vitamin D status increases cancer risk and whether higher levels protect or even increase risk in some people.

Can Vitamin D Be Harmful?

Yes, when amounts in the blood become too high. Signs of toxicity include nausea, vomiting, poor appetite, constipation, weakness, and weight loss. And by raising blood levels of calcium, too much vitamin D can cause confusion, disorientation, and problems with heart rhythm. Excess vitamin D can also damage the kidneys.

The upper limit for vitamin D is 1,000 to 1,500 IU/day for infants, 2,500 to 3,000 IU/day for children 1–8 years, and 4,000 IU/day for children 9 years and older, adults, and pregnant and lactating teens and women. Vitamin D toxicity almost always occurs from overuse of supplements. Excessive sun exposure doesn't cause vitamin D poisoning because the body limits the amount of this vitamin it produces.

Chapter 16
Vitamin E

What Is Vitamin E And What Does It Do?

Vitamin E is a fat-soluble nutrient found in many foods. In the body, it acts as an antioxidant, helping to protect cells from the damage caused by free radicals. Free radicals are compounds formed when our bodies convert the food we eat into energy. People are also exposed to free radicals in the environment from cigarette smoke, air pollution, and ultraviolet light from the sun.

The body also needs vitamin E to boost its immune system so that it can fight off invading bacteria and viruses. It helps to widen blood vessels and keep blood from clotting within them. In addition, cells use vitamin E to interact with each other and to carry out many important functions.

How Much Vitamin E Do I Need?

The amount of vitamin E you need each day depends on your age. Average daily recommended intake is listed below in milligrams (mg) and in International Units (IU). Package labels list the amount of vitamin E in foods and dietary supplements in IU.

Table 16.1. Average Daily Recommended Intake Of Vitamin E

Life Stage	Recommended Amount
Teens 14–18 years	15 mg (22.4 IU)

About This Chapter: Information in this chapter is excerpted from "Vitamin E Fact Sheet for Consumers," Office on Dietary Supplements (ODS), National Institutes of Health (NIH), May 9, 2016.

What Foods Provide Vitamin E?

Vitamin E is found naturally in foods and is added to some fortified foods. You can get recommended amounts of vitamin E by eating a variety of foods including the following:

- Vegetable oils like wheat germ, sunflower, and safflower oils are among the best sources of vitamin E. Corn and soybean oils also provide some vitamin E.
- Nuts (such as peanuts, hazelnuts, and, especially, almonds) and seeds (like sunflower seeds) are also among the best sources of vitamin E.
- Green vegetables, such as spinach and broccoli, provide some vitamin E.
- Food companies add vitamin E to some breakfast cereals, fruit juices, margarines and spreads, and other foods. To find out which ones have vitamin E, check the product labels.

What Kinds Of Vitamin E Dietary Supplements Are Available?

Vitamin E supplements come in different amounts and forms. Two main things to consider when choosing a vitamin E supplement are:

1. *The amount of vitamin E*: Most once-daily multivitamin-mineral supplements provide about 30 IU of vitamin E, whereas vitamin E-only supplements usually contain 100 to 1,000 IU per pill. The doses in vitamin E-only supplements are much higher than the recommended amounts. Some people take large doses because they believe or hope that doing so will keep them healthy or lower their risk of certain diseases.

2. *The form of vitamin E*: Although vitamin E sounds like a single substance, it is actually the name of eight related compounds in food, including alpha-tocopherol. Each form has a different potency, or level of activity in the body.

Vitamin E from natural (food) sources is commonly listed as "*d*-alpha-tocopherol" on food packaging and supplement labels. Synthetic (laboratory-made) vitamin E is commonly listed as "*dl*-alpha-tocopherol." The natural form is more potent. For example, 100 IU of natural vitamin E is equal to about 150 IU of the synthetic form.

Some vitamin E supplements provide other forms of the vitamin, such as gamma-tocopherol, tocotrienols, and mixed tocopherols. Scientists do not know if any of these forms are superior to alpha-tocopherol in supplements.

What Are Some Effects Of Vitamin E On Health?

Scientists are studying vitamin E to understand how it affects health. Here are several examples of what this research has shown.

Heart Disease

Some studies link higher intakes of vitamin E from supplements to lower chances of developing heart disease. But the best research finds no benefit. People in these studies are randomly assigned to take vitamin E or a placebo (dummy pill with no vitamin E or active ingredients) and they don't know which they are taking. Vitamin E supplements do not seem to prevent heart disease, reduce its severity, or affect the risk of death from this disease. Scientists do not know whether high intakes of vitamin E might protect the heart in younger, healthier people who do not have a high risk of heart disease.

Cancer

Most research indicates that vitamin E does not help prevent cancer and may be harmful in some cases. Large doses of vitamin E have not consistently reduced the risk of colon and breast cancer in studies, for example. A large study found that taking vitamin E supplements (400 IU/day) for several years increased the risk of developing prostate cancer in men. Two studies that followed middle-aged men and women for 7 or more years found that extra vitamin E (300–400 IU/day, on average) did not protect them from any form of cancer. However, one study found a link between the use of vitamin E supplements for 10 years or more and a lower risk of death from bladder cancer.

Vitamin E dietary supplements and other antioxidants might interact with chemotherapy and radiation therapy. People undergoing these treatments should talk with their doctor or oncologist before taking vitamin E or other antioxidant supplements, especially in high doses.

Eye Disorders

Age-related macular degeneration (AMD), or the loss of central vision in older people, and cataracts are among the most common causes of vision loss in older people. The results of research on whether vitamin E can help prevent these conditions are inconsistent. Among people with AMD who were at high risk of developing advanced AMD, a supplement containing large doses of vitamin E combined with other antioxidants, zinc, and copper showed promise for slowing down the rate of vision loss.

Mental Function

Several studies have investigated whether vitamin E supplements might help older adults remain mentally alert and active as well as prevent or slow the decline of mental function and Alzheimer's disease. So far, the research provides little evidence that taking vitamin E supplements can help healthy people or people with mild mental functioning problems to maintain brain health.

Can Vitamin E Be Harmful?

Eating vitamin E in foods is not risky or harmful.

In supplement form, however, high doses of vitamin E might increase the risk of bleeding (by reducing the blood's ability to form clots after a cut or injury) and of serious bleeding in the brain (known as hemorrhagic stroke). Because of this risk, the upper limit for adults is 1,500 IU/day for supplements made from the natural form of vitamin E and 1,100 IU/day for supplements made from synthetic vitamin E. The upper limits for children are lower than those for adults. Some research suggests that taking vitamin E supplements even below these upper limits might cause harm.

In one study, for example, men who took 400 IU of vitamin E each day for several years had an increased risk of prostate cancer.

Chapter 17
Vitamin K

What Is Vitamin K And What Does It Do?

Vitamin K is a nutrient that the body needs to stay healthy. It's important for blood clotting and healthy bones and also has other functions in the body. If you are taking a blood thinner such as warfarin (Coumadin®), it's very important to get about the same amount of vitamin K each day.

How Much Vitamin K Do I Need?

The amount of vitamin K you need depends on your age and sex. Average daily recommended amount is listed below in micrograms (mcg).

Table 17.1. Average Daily Recommended Intake Of Vitamin K

Life Stage	Recommended Amount
Teens 14–18 years	75 mcg

What Foods Provide Vitamin K?

Vitamin K is found naturally in many foods. You can get recommended amounts of vitamin K by eating a variety of foods, including the following:

- green leafy vegetables, such as spinach, kale, broccoli, and lettuce
- vegetable oils
- some fruits, such as blueberries and figs
- meat, cheese, eggs, and soybeans

About This Chapter: Information in this chapter is excerpted from "Vitamin K," Office on Dietary Supplements (ODS), National Institutes of Health (NIH), April 13, 2016.

What Kinds Of Vitamin K Dietary Supplements Are Available?

Vitamin K is found in multivitamin/multimineral supplements. Vitamin K is also available in supplements of vitamin K alone or of vitamin K with a few other nutrients such as calcium, magnesium, and/or vitamin D. Common forms of vitamin K in dietary supplements are phylloquinone and phytonadione (also called vitamin K1), menaquinone-4, and menaquinone-7 (also called vitamin K2).

Am I Getting Enough Vitamin K?

Vitamin K deficiency is very rare. Most people in the United States get enough vitamin K from the foods they eat. Also, bacteria in the colon make some vitamin K that the body can absorb. However, certain groups of people may have trouble getting enough vitamin K:

- Newborns who don't receive an injection of vitamin K at birth

- People with conditions (such as cystic fibrosis, celiac disease, ulcerative colitis, and short bowel syndrome) that decrease the amount of vitamin K their body absorbs

- People who have had bariatric (weight loss) surgery

What Happens If I Don't Get Enough Vitamin K?

Severe vitamin K deficiency can cause bruising and bleeding problems because the blood will take longer to clot. Vitamin K deficiency might reduce bone strength and increase the risk of getting osteoporosis because the body needs vitamin K for healthy bones.

What Are Some Effects Of Vitamin K On Health?

Scientists are studying vitamin K to understand how it affects our health. Here are some examples of what this research has shown.

Osteoporosis

Vitamin K is important for healthy bones. Some research shows that people who eat more vitamin K-rich foods have stronger bones and are less likely to break a hip than those who eat less of these foods. A few studies have found that taking vitamin K supplements improves bone strength and the chances of breaking a bone, but other studies have not. More research is needed to better understand if vitamin K supplements can help improve bone health and reduce osteoporosis risk.

Coronary Heart Disease

Scientists are studying whether low blood levels of vitamin K increase the risk of heart disease, perhaps by making blood vessels that feed the heart stiffer and narrower. More research is needed to understand whether vitamin K supplements might help prevent heart disease.

Can Vitamin K Be Harmful?

Vitamin K has not been shown to cause any harm. However, it can interact with some medications, particularly warfarin (Coumadin®).

Chapter 18
Calcium

What Is Calcium and How Does It Build Strong Bones?

Calcium is a mineral that helps bones stay strong. Our bodies continually remove small amounts of calcium from our bones and replace it with new calcium, a bone "remodeling" process. If the body removes more calcium from bones than it replaces, they slowly become weaker and more prone to breaking. Eating a diet rich in calcium allows the body to deposit calcium in bones so they stay strong.

Children and teens who eat calcium-rich foods build up stores of calcium in their bones that help them maintain strong bones for life. By getting lots of calcium when you're young, you can make sure your body doesn't have to take too much from your bones. Bones have their own "calcium bank account," so "depositing" as much calcium as possible during your tween and teen years will help you reach your peak bone mass. By the end of the teen years, the account "closes"—you can't add any more calcium to your bones. You can only maintain what is already stored to help your bones stay healthy.

How Much Calcium Do I Need?

The amount of calcium you need each day depends on your age. Average daily recommended amount is listed below in milligrams (mg):

About This Chapter: Information in this chapter is excerpted from "Calcium," Office on Dietary Supplements (ODS), National Institutes of Health (NIH), June 1, 2016; and information from "Children's Bone Health and Calcium," *Eunice Kennedy Shriver* National Institute of Child Health and Human Development (NICHD), May 6, 2014.

Table 18.1. Average Daily Recommended Amount Of Calcium

Life Stage	Recommended Amount
Teens 14–18 years	1,300 mg

Many children and teens do not get enough calcium. One large survey found that among children aged 9 to 13 years, only about 12 percent of girls and 17 percent of boys consumed the recommended daily amount of calcium. For older teens, 42 percent of boys and only 10 percent of girls consumed enough calcium daily.

What Are Good Sources of Calcium?

Dairy Sources

A variety of foods contain calcium. Milk and other dairy products contain a lot of calcium. Low-fat and fat-free milk and dairy products are also great sources of calcium because:

- They contain little or no fat.

- The calcium in low-fat and fat-free milk and dairy products is easy for the body to absorb.

- Low-fat and fat-free milk have added vitamin D, which helps the body absorb the calcium.

- Milk and dairy products also provide other essential nutrients that are important for optimal bone health and development.

Tweens and teens can get most of their daily calcium by drinking 3 cups of low-fat or fat-free milk, but they do need additional calcium (400 mg more) to get the entire 1,300 mg that is necessary for strong bone growth. Other good sources of calcium include milk products and milk substitutes, such as:

- Flavored milk (for example, chocolate milk)

- Lactose-free or lactose-reduced milk

- Buttermilk

- Plain or fruit yogurt

- Cheese

- Rice milk or soy milk with added calcium

Nondairy Sources

Milk isn't the only way for tweens and teens to get the 1,300 mg calcium they need every day. This is especially important for people who have lactose intolerance or who don't eat dairy products. Other good sources of calcium include:

- Dark green, leafy vegetables (such as spinach, broccoli, and bok choy)

- Some fish

- Several servings of vegetables (to get the amount of calcium in a cup of milk)

Foods that are fortified with calcium (calcium is added) are also a good option. Check the ingredient list for:

- Tofu (with added calcium sulfate)

- Calcium-fortified orange juice

- Soy beverages with added calcium

- Calcium-fortified cereals or breads

Calcium supplements are an additional, alternative way to get calcium for children and adults who do not drink or cannot have milk or milk products.

Food labels on packaged, bottled, and canned foods show how much calcium is in one serving of food. Look at the % Daily Value (or %DV) next to the calcium number on the food label.

The following chart lists selected food sources ranked by the approximate amount of calcium in a standard portion:

Table 18.2. Calcium Amounts In A Standard Portion

Food	Portion Size	Calcium (mg)
Yogurt, plain, low fat	8 oz	415
Orange juice, calcium fortified	6 oz	375
Yogurt, fruit, low fat	8 oz	338–384
Mozzarella cheese, part skim	1½ oz	333
Sardines, canned in oil, with bones	3 oz	325
Cheddar cheese	1½ oz	307
Milk, nonfat	8 oz	299
Milk, reduced fat (2% milk fat)	8 oz	293
Milk, buttermilk	8 oz	282–350

Table 18.2. Continued

Food	Portion Size	Calcium (mg)
Milk, whole (3.25% milk fat)	8 oz	276
Tofu, firm, made with calcium	4 oz	253
Salmon, pink, canned, solids with bone	3 oz	181
Cottage cheese (1% milk fat)	8 oz	138
Tofu, soft, made with calcium sulfate	4 oz	138
Instant breakfast drink, powder prepared with water	8 oz	105–250
Frozen yogurt, vanilla, soft serve	4 oz	103
Ready-to-eat cereal, calcium fortified	8 oz	100–1,000
Turnip greens, fresh, boiled	4 oz	99
Kale, fresh, cooked	8 oz	94
Kale, raw, chopped	8 oz	90
Ice cream, vanilla	4 oz	84
Soy milk, calcium fortified	8 oz	80–500
Chinese cabbage (bok choy), raw, shredded	8 oz	74
Bread, white	1 slice	73
Broccoli, raw	8 oz	21

What Kinds Of Calcium Dietary Supplements Are Available?

Calcium is found in many multivitamin-mineral supplements, though the amount varies by product. Dietary supplements that contain only calcium or calcium with other nutrients such as vitamin D are also available. Check the Supplement Facts label to determine the amount of calcium provided.

The two main forms of calcium dietary supplements are carbonate and citrate. Calcium carbonate is inexpensive, but is absorbed best when taken with food. Some over-the-counter antacid products, such as Tums® and Rolaids®, contain calcium carbonate. Each pill or chew provides 200–400 mg of calcium. Calcium citrate, a more expensive form of the supplement, is absorbed well on an empty or a full stomach. In addition, people with low levels of stomach acid (a condition more common in people older than 50) absorb calcium citrate more easily than calcium carbonate. Other forms of calcium in supplements and fortified foods include gluconate, lactate, and phosphate.

Calcium absorption is best when a person consumes no more than 500 mg at one time. So a person who takes 1,000 mg/day of calcium from supplements, for example, should split the dose rather than take it all at once.

Calcium supplements may cause gas, bloating, and constipation in some people. If any of these symptoms occur, try spreading out the calcium dose throughout the day, taking the supplement with meals, or changing the supplement brand or calcium form you take.

What Are Some Effects Of Calcium On Health?

Scientists are studying calcium to understand how it affects health. Here are several examples of what this research has shown:

Bone Health And Osteoporosis

Bones need plenty of calcium and vitamin D throughout childhood and adolescence to reach their peak strength and calcium content by about age 30. After that, bones slowly lose calcium, but people can help reduce these losses by getting recommended amounts of calcium throughout adulthood and by having a healthy, active lifestyle that includes weight-bearing physical activity (such as walking and running).

Osteoporosis is a disease of the bones in older adults (especially women) in which the bones become porous, fragile, and more prone to fracture. Osteoporosis is a serious public health problem for more than 10 million adults over the age of 50 in the United States. Adequate calcium and vitamin D intakes as well as regular exercise are essential to keep bones healthy throughout life.

Taking calcium and vitamin D supplements reduce the risk of breaking a bone and the risk of falling in frail, elderly adults who live in nursing homes and similar facilities. But it's not clear if the supplements help prevent bone fractures and falls in older people who live at home.

Cancer

Studies have examined whether calcium supplements or diets high in calcium might lower the risks of developing cancer of the colon or rectum or increase the risk of prostate cancer. The research to date provides no clear answers. Given that cancer develops over many years, longer term studies are needed.

Cardiovascular Disease

Whether calcium affects the risk of cardiovascular disease is not clear. Some studies show that getting enough calcium might protect people from heart disease and stroke. But other studies show that some people who consume high amounts of calcium, particularly from supplements, might have an increased risk of heart disease. More research is needed in this area.

High Blood Pressure

Some studies have found that getting recommended intakes of calcium can reduce the risk of developing high blood pressure (hypertension). One large study in particular found that eating a diet high in fat-free and low-fat dairy products, vegetables, and fruits lowered blood pressure.

Kidney Stones

Most kidney stones are rich in calcium oxalate. Some studies have found that higher intakes of calcium from dietary supplements are linked to a greater risk of kidney stones, especially among older adults. But calcium from foods does not appear to cause kidney stones. For most people, other factors (such as not drinking enough fluids) probably have a larger effect on the risk of kidney stones than calcium intake.

Weight Loss

Although several studies have shown that getting more calcium helps lower body weight or reduce weight gain over time, most studies have found that calcium—from foods or dietary supplements—has little if any effect on body weight and amount of body fat.

Can Calcium Be Harmful?

Getting too much calcium can cause constipation. It might also interfere with the body's ability to absorb iron and zinc, but this effect is not well established. In adults, too much calcium (from dietary supplements but not food) might increase the risk of kidney stones. Some studies show that people who consume high amounts of calcium might have increased risks of prostate cancer and heart disease, but more research is needed to understand these possible links.

The upper limit for calcium is listed below. Most people do not get amounts above the upper limits from food alone; excess intakes usually come from the use of calcium supplements.

Table 18.3. The Upper Limit For Calcium

Life Stage	Upper Limit
9–18 years	3,000 mg

Chapter 19
Iron

What Is Iron And What Does It Do?

Iron is a mineral that the body needs for growth and development. Your body uses iron to make hemoglobin, a protein in red blood cells that carries oxygen from the lungs to all parts of the body, and myoglobin, a protein that provides oxygen to muscles. Your body also needs iron to make some hormones and connective tissue.

How Much Iron Do I Need?

The amount of iron you need each day depends on your age, your sex, and whether you consume a mostly plant-based diet. Average daily recommended amounts are listed below in milligrams (mg). Vegetarians who do not eat meat, poultry, or seafood need almost twice as much iron as listed in the table because the body doesn't absorb non-heme iron in plant foods as well as heme iron in animal foods.

Table 19.1. Average Daily Recommended Amounts Of Iron

Life Stage	Recommended Amount
Teens boys 14–18 years	11 mg
Teens girls 14–18 years	15 mg
Breastfeeding teens	10 mg

About This Chapter: Information in this chapter is excerpted from "Iron," Office on Dietary Supplements (ODS), National Institutes of Health (NIH), February 17, 2016.

What Foods Provide Iron?

Iron is found naturally in many foods and is added to some fortified food products. You can get recommended amounts of iron by eating a variety of foods, including the following:

- Lean meat, seafood, and poultry.
- Iron-fortified breakfast cereals and breads.
- White beans, lentils, spinach, kidney beans, and peas.
- Nuts and some dried fruits, such as raisins.

Iron in food comes in two forms: heme iron and non-heme iron. Non-heme iron is found in plant foods and iron-fortified food products. Meat, seafood, and poultry have both heme and non-heme iron.

Your body absorbs iron from plant sources better when you eat it with meat, poultry, seafood, and foods that contain vitamin C, like citrus fruits, strawberries, sweet peppers, tomatoes, and broccoli.

What Kinds Of Iron Dietary Supplements Are Available?

Iron is available in many multivitamin-mineral supplements and in supplements that contain only iron. Iron in supplements is often in the form of ferrous sulfate, ferrous gluconate, ferric citrate, or ferric sulfate. Dietary supplements that contain iron have a statement on the label warning that they should be kept out of the reach of children. Accidental overdose of iron-containing products is a leading cause of fatal poisoning in children under 6.

Am I Getting Enough Iron?

Most people in the United States get enough iron. However, certain groups of people are more likely than others to have trouble getting enough iron:

- Teen girls and women with heavy periods.
- Pregnant women and teens.
- Frequent blood donors.
- People with cancer, gastrointestinal (GI) disorders, or heart failure.

What Happens If I Don't Get Enough Iron?

In the short term, getting too little iron does not cause obvious symptoms. The body uses its stored iron in the muscles, liver, spleen, and bone marrow. But when levels of iron stored in the body become low, iron deficiency anemia sets in. Red blood cells become smaller and contain less hemoglobin. As a result, blood carries less oxygen from the lungs throughout the body.

Symptoms of iron deficiency anemia include tiredness and lack of energy, GI upset, poor memory and concentration, and less ability to fight off germs and infections or to control body temperature. Infants and children with iron deficiency anemia might develop learning difficulties.

Iron deficiency is not common in the United States. But it can occur in people who do not eat meat, poultry, or seafood; lose blood; have GI diseases that interfere with nutrient absorption; or eat poor diets.

What Are Some Effects Of Iron On Health?

Scientists are studying iron to understand how it affects health. Iron's most important contribution to health is preventing iron deficiency anemia and resulting problems.

Pregnant Women

During pregnancy, the amount of blood in a woman's body increases, so she needs more iron for herself and her growing baby. Getting too little iron during pregnancy increases a woman's risk of iron deficiency anemia and her infant's risk of low birthweight, premature birth, and low levels of iron. Getting too little iron might also harm her infant's brain development.

Women who are pregnant or breastfeeding should take an iron supplement as recommended by an obstetrician or other healthcare provider.

Anemia Of Chronic Disease

Some chronic diseases—like rheumatoid arthritis, inflammatory bowel disease, and some types of cancer—can interfere with the body's ability to use its stored iron. Taking more iron from foods or supplements usually does not reduce the resulting anemia of chronic disease because iron is diverted from the blood circulation to storage sites. The main therapy for anemia of chronic disease is treatment of the underlying disease.

Can Iron Be Harmful?

Yes, iron can be harmful if you get too much. In healthy people, taking high doses of iron supplements (especially on an empty stomach) can cause an upset stomach, constipation, nausea, abdominal pain, vomiting, and fainting. High doses of iron can also decrease zinc absorption. Extremely high doses of iron (in the hundreds or thousands of mg) can cause organ failure, coma, convulsions, and death. Child-proof packaging and warning labels on iron supplements have greatly reduced the number of accidental iron poisonings in children.

Some people have an inherited condition called hemochromatosis that causes toxic levels of iron to build up in their bodies. Without medical treatment, people with hereditary hemochromatosis can develop serious problems like liver cirrhosis, liver cancer, and heart disease. People with this disorder should avoid using iron supplements and vitamin C supplements.

The upper limits for iron from foods and dietary supplements are listed below. A doctor might prescribe more than the upper limit of iron to people who need higher doses for a while to treat iron deficiency.

Table 19.2. The Upper Limits For Iron From Foods And Dietary Supplements

Ages	Upper Limit
Children 1–13 years	40 mg
Teens 14–18 years	45 mg

Chapter 20
Magnesium

What Is Magnesium And What Does It Do?

Magnesium is a nutrient that the body needs to stay healthy. Magnesium is important for many processes in the body, including regulating muscle and nerve function, blood sugar levels, and blood pressure and making protein, bone, and DNA.

What Happens If I Don't Get Enough Magnesium?

When healthy people have low intakes, the kidneys help retain magnesium by limiting the amount lost in urine. Low magnesium intakes for a long period of time, however, can lead to magnesium deficiency.

How Much Magnesium Do I Need?

The amount of magnesium you need depends on your age and sex. Average daily recommended amounts are listed below in milligrams (mg):

Table 20.1. Average Daily Recommended Amounts Of Magnesium

Life Stage	Recommended Amount
Teen boys 14–18 years	410 mg
Teen girls 14–18 years	360 mg
Pregnant teens	400 mg
Breastfeeding teens	360 mg

About This Chapter: Information in this chapter is excerpted from "Magnesium," Office on Dietary Supplements (ODS), National Institutes of Health (NIH), February 17, 2016.

What Foods Provide Magnesium?

Magnesium is found naturally in many foods and is added to some fortified foods. You can get recommended amounts of magnesium by eating a variety of foods, including the following:

- legumes, nuts, seeds, whole grains, and green leafy vegetables (such as spinach)
- fortified breakfast cereals and other fortified foods
- milk, yogurt, and some other milk products

What Kinds Of Magnesium Dietary Supplements Are Available?

Magnesium is available in multivitamin-mineral supplements and other dietary supplements. Forms of magnesium in dietary supplements that are more easily absorbed by the body are magnesium aspartate, magnesium citrate, magnesium lactate, and magnesium chloride.

Magnesium is also included in some laxatives and some products for treating heartburn and indigestion.

What Are Some Effects Of Magnesium On Health?

Scientists are studying magnesium to understand how it affects health. Here are some examples of what this research has shown.

High Blood Pressure And Heart Disease

High blood pressure is a major risk factor for heart disease and stroke. Magnesium supplements might decrease blood pressure, but only by a small amount. Some studies show that people who have more magnesium in their diets have a lower risk of some types of heart disease and stroke. But in many of these studies, it's hard to know how much of the effect was due to magnesium as opposed to other nutrients.

Type 2 Diabetes

People with higher amounts of magnesium in their diets tend to have a lower risk of developing type 2 diabetes. Magnesium helps the body break down sugars and might help reduce the risk of insulin resistance (a condition that leads to diabetes). Scientists are studying whether magnesium supplements might help people who already have type 2 diabetes control their disease. More research is needed to better understand whether magnesium can help treat diabetes.

Osteoporosis

Magnesium is important for healthy bones. People with higher intakes of magnesium have a higher bone mineral density, which is important in reducing the risk of bone fractures and osteoporosis. Getting more magnesium from foods or dietary supplements might help older women improve their bone mineral density. More research is needed to better understand whether magnesium supplements can help reduce the risk of osteoporosis or treat this condition.

Migraine Headaches

People who have migraine headaches sometimes have low levels of magnesium in their blood and other tissues. Several small studies found that magnesium supplements can modestly reduce the frequency of migraines. However, people should only take magnesium for this purpose under the care of a healthcare provider. More research is needed to determine whether magnesium supplements can help reduce the risk of migraines or ease migraine symptoms.

Can Magnesium Be Harmful?

Magnesium that is naturally present in food is not harmful and does not need to be limited. In healthy people, the kidneys can get rid of any excess in the urine. But magnesium in dietary supplements and medications should not be consumed in amounts above the upper limit, unless recommended by a healthcare provider.

The upper limit for magnesium from dietary supplements and/or medications is listed below. For many age groups, the upper limit appears to be lower than the recommended amount. This occurs because the recommended amounts include magnesium from **all** sources—food, dietary supplements and medications. The upper limit includes magnesium from **only** dietary supplements and medications; it does **not** include magnesium found naturally in food.

Table 20.2. The Upper Limits For Magnesium From Dietary Supplements And/ Or Medications

Ages	Upper Limit for Magnesium in Dietary Supplements and Medications
Children and Teens 9–18 years	350 mg

Chapter 21
Zinc

What Is Zinc And What Does It Do?

Zinc is a nutrient that people need to stay healthy. Zinc is found in cells throughout the body. It helps the immune system fight off invading bacteria and viruses. The body also needs zinc to make proteins and DNA, the genetic material in all cells. During pregnancy, infancy, and childhood, the body needs zinc to grow and develop properly. Zinc also helps wounds heal and is important for proper senses of taste and smell.

What Happens If I Don't Get Enough Zinc?

Zinc deficiency causes slow growth in children and delayed sexual development in adolescents. Zinc deficiency also causes hair loss, diarrhea, eye and skin sores and loss of appetite.

How Much Zinc Do I Need?

The amount of zinc you need each day depends on your age. Average daily recommended amounts for different ages are listed below in milligrams (mg):

Table 21.1. Average Daily Recommended Amounts Of Zinc

Life Stage	Recommended Amount
Teens 14–18 years (boys)	11 mg
Teens 14–18 years (girls)	9 mg

About This Chapter: Information in this chapter is excerpted from "Zinc," Office on Dietary Supplements (ODS), National Institutes of Health (NIH), February 17, 2016.

What Foods Provide Zinc?

Zinc is found in a wide variety of foods. You can get recommended amounts of zinc by eating a variety of foods including the following:

- oysters, which are the best source of zinc
- red meat, poultry, seafood such as crab and lobsters, and fortified breakfast cereals, which are also good sources of zinc
- beans, nuts, whole grains, and dairy products, which provide some zinc

---

What Kinds Of Zinc Dietary Supplements Are Available?

Zinc is present in almost all multivitamin/mineral dietary supplements. It is also available alone or combined with calcium, magnesium or other ingredients in dietary supplements. Dietary supplements can have several different forms of zinc including zinc gluconate, zinc sulfate and zinc acetate. It is not clear whether one form is better than the others.

Zinc is also found in some oral over-the-counter products, including those labeled as homeopathic medications for colds. Use of nasal sprays and gels that contain zinc has been associated with the loss of the sense of smell, in some cases long-lasting or permanent. Currently, these safety concerns have not been found to be associated with oral products containing zinc, such as cold lozenges.

Zinc is also present in some denture adhesive creams. Using large amounts of these products, well beyond recommended levels, could lead to excessive zinc intake and copper deficiency. This can cause neurological problems, including numbness and weakness in the arms and legs.

What Are Some Effects Of Zinc On Health?

Scientists are studying zinc to learn about its effects on the immune system (the body's defense system against bacteria, viruses, and other foreign invaders). Scientists are also researching possible connections between zinc and the health problems discussed below.

Immune System And Wound Healing

The body's immune system needs zinc to do its job. Older people and children in developing countries who have low levels of zinc might have a higher risk of getting pneumonia and other infections. Zinc also helps the skin stay healthy. Some people who have skin ulcers might benefit from zinc dietary supplements, but only if they have low levels of zinc.

Diarrhea

Children in developing countries often die from diarrhea. Studies show that zinc dietary supplements help reduce the symptoms and duration of diarrhea in these children, many of whom are zinc deficient or otherwise malnourished. The World Health Organization and UNICEF recommend that children with diarrhea take zinc for 10–14 days (20 mg/day, or 10 mg/day for infants under 6 months). It is not clear whether zinc dietary supplements can help treat diarrhea in children who get enough zinc, such as most children in the United States.

The Common Cold

Some studies suggest that zinc lozenges or syrup (but not zinc dietary supplements in pill form) help speed recovery from the common cold and reduce its symptoms if taken within 24 hours of coming down with a cold. However, more study is needed to determine the best dose and form of zinc, as well as how long it should be taken before zinc can be recommended as a treatment for the common cold.

Age-Related Macular Degeneration (AMD)

AMD is an eye disease that gradually causes vision loss. Research suggests that zinc might help slow AMD progression. In a large study among older people with AMD who were at high risk of developing advanced AMD, those who took a daily dietary supplement with 80 mg zinc, 500 mg vitamin C, 400 IU vitamin E, 15 mg beta-carotene, and 2 mg copper for about 6 years had a lower chance of developing advanced AMD and less vision loss than those who did not take the dietary supplement. In the same study, people at high risk of the disease who took dietary supplements containing only zinc also had a lower risk of getting advanced AMD than those who did not take zinc dietary supplements. People who have or are developing the disease might want to talk with their doctor about taking dietary supplements.

Can Zinc Be Harmful?

Yes, if you get too much. Signs of too much zinc include nausea, vomiting, loss of appetite, stomach cramps, diarrhea, and headaches. When people take too much zinc for a long time, they sometimes have problems such as low copper levels, lower immunity, and low levels of HDL cholesterol (the "good" cholesterol).

The upper limit for zinc is listed below. This level does not apply to people who are taking zinc for medical reasons under the care of a doctor:

Table 21.2. The Upper Limit For Zinc

Life Stage	Upper Limit
Teens 14–18 years	34 mg

Chapter 22
Other Important Minerals

Chromium

What Is It?

Chromium is a mineral that humans require in trace amounts, although its mechanisms of action in the body and the amounts needed for optimal health are not well defined. It is found primarily in two forms:

1. trivalent (chromium 3+), which is biologically active and found in food, and

2. hexavalent (chromium 6+), a toxic form that results from industrial pollution.

This chapter focuses exclusively on trivalent (3+) chromium.

Chromium is known to enhance the action of insulin, a hormone critical to the metabolism and storage of carbohydrate, fat, and protein in the body. In 1957, a compound in brewers' yeast was found to prevent an age-related decline in the ability of rats to maintain normal levels of sugar (glucose) in their blood. Chromium was identified as the active ingredient in this so-called "glucose tolerance factor" in 1959.

Chromium also appears to be directly involved in carbohydrate, fat, and protein metabolism, but more research is needed to determine the full range of its roles in the body.

About This Chapter: Information in this chapter is excerpted from "Chromium," Office of Dietary Supplements (ODS), National Institutes of Health (NIH), November 4, 2013; and information from "Selenium," Office of Dietary Supplements (ODS), National Institutes of Health (NIH), February 11, 2016.

What Foods Provide Chromium?

Chromium is widely distributed in the food supply, but most foods provide only small amounts (less than 2 micrograms [mcg] per serving). Meat and whole-grain products, as well as some fruits, vegetables, and spices are relatively good sources. In contrast, foods high in simple sugars (like sucrose and fructose) are low in chromium.

Dietary intakes of chromium cannot be reliably determined because the content of the mineral in foods is substantially affected by agricultural and manufacturing processes and perhaps by contamination with chromium when the foods are analyzed. Therefore, Table 22.1., and food-composition databases generally, provide approximate values of chromium in foods that should only serve as a guide.

Table 22.1. Selected Food Sources Of Chromium

Food	Chromium (mcg)
Broccoli, ½ cup	11
Grape juice, 1 cup	8
English muffin, whole wheat, 1	4
Potatoes, mashed, 1 cup	3
Garlic, dried, 1 teaspoon	3
Basil, dried, 1 tablespoon	2
Beef cubes, 3 ounces	2
Orange juice, 1 cup	2
Turkey breast, 3 ounces	2
Whole wheat bread, 2 slices	2
Red wine, 5 ounces	1–13
Apple, unpeeled, 1 medium	1
Banana, 1 medium	1
Green beans, ½ cup	1

What Are Recommended Intakes Of Chromium?

Recommended chromium intakes are provided in the Dietary Reference Intakes (DRIs) developed by the Institute of Medicine of the National Academy of Sciences. *Dietary Reference Intakes* is the general term for a set of reference values to plan and assess the nutrient intakes of healthy people. These values include the *Recommended Dietary Allowance* (RDA) and the *Adequate Intake* (AI). The RDA is the average daily intake that meets a nutrient requirement of nearly all (97 to 98%) healthy individuals. An AI is established when there is insufficient research to establish an RDA; it is generally set at a level that healthy people typically consume.

Table 22.2. Adequate Intakes (AIs) For Chromium

Age	Males (mcg/day)	Females (mcg/day)	Pregnancy (mcg/day)	Lactation (mcg/day)
9 to 13 years	25	21		
14 to 18 years	35	24	29	44

What Affects Chromium Levels In The Body?

Absorption of chromium from the intestinal tract is low, ranging from less than 0.4% to 2.5% of the amount consumed, and the remainder is excreted in the feces. Enhancing the mineral's absorption are vitamin C (found in fruits and vegetables and their juices) and the B vitamin niacin (found in meats, poultry, fish, and grain products). Absorbed chromium is stored in the liver, spleen, soft tissue, and bone.

The body's chromium content may be reduced under several conditions. Diets high in simple sugars (comprising more than 35% of calories) can increase chromium excretion in the urine. Infection, acute exercise, pregnancy and lactation, and stressful states (such as physical trauma) increase chromium losses and can lead to deficiency, especially if chromium intakes are already low.

Who May Need Extra Chromium?

There are reports of significant age-related decreases in the chromium concentrations of hair, sweat and blood. One cannot be sure, however, as chromium status is difficult to determine. That's because blood, urine, and hair levels do not necessarily reflect body stores. Furthermore, no chromium-specific enzyme or other biochemical marker has been found to reliably assess a person's chromium status.

There is considerable interest in the possibility that supplemental chromium may help to treat impaired glucose tolerance and type 2 diabetes, but the research to date is inconclusive. No large, randomized, controlled clinical trials testing this hypothesis have been reported in the United States. Nevertheless, this is an active area of research.

Chromium And Medication Interactions

Certain medications may interact with chromium, especially when taken on a regular basis (see Table 22.3.). Before taking dietary supplements, check with your doctor or other qualified healthcare provider, especially if you take prescription or over-the-counter medications.

Table 22.3. Interactions between Chromium and Medications

Medications	Nature of interaction
• Antacids • Corticosteroids • H2 blockers (such as cimetidine, famotidine, nizatidine, and rantidine) • Proton-pump inhibitors (such as omeprazole, lansoprazole, rabeprazole, pantoprazole, and esomeprazole)	These medications alter stomach acidity and may impair chromium absorption or enhance excretion
• Beta-blockers (such as atenolol or propano-lol) • Corticosteroids • Insulin • Nicotinic acid • Nonsteroidal anti-inflammatory drugs (NSAIDS) • Prostaglandin inhibitors (such as ibuprofen, indomethacin, naproxen, piroxicam, and aspirin)	These medications may have their effects enhanced if taken together with chromium or they may increase chromium absorption

Supplemental Sources Of Chromium

Chromium is a widely used supplement. Estimated sales to consumers were $85 million in 2002, representing 5.6% of the total mineral-supplement market. Chromium is sold as a single-ingredient supplement as well as in combination formulas, particularly those marketed for weight loss and performance enhancement. Supplement doses typically range from 50 to 200 mcg.

The safety and efficacy of chromium supplements need more investigation. Please consult with a doctor or other trained healthcare professional before taking any dietary supplements.

Chromium And Healthful Diets

The federal government's 2015–2020 Dietary Guidelines for Americans notes that "Nutritional needs should be met primarily from foods. ... Foods in nutrient-dense forms contain essential vitamins and minerals and also dietary fiber and other naturally occurring substances that may have positive health effects. In some cases, fortified foods and dietary supplements may be useful in providing one or more nutrients that otherwise may be consumed in less-than-recommended amounts."

Selenium

What Is Selenium And What Does It Do?

Selenium is a nutrient that the body needs to stay healthy. Selenium is important for reproduction, thyroid gland function, DNA production, and protecting the body from damage caused by free radicals and from infection.

How Much Selenium Do I Need?

The amount of selenium that you need each day depends on your age. Average daily recommended amount is listed below in micrograms (mcg).

Table 22.4. Life Stage with Recommended Amount

Life Stage	Recommended Amount
Teens 14–18 years	55 mcg

What Foods Provide Selenium?

Selenium is found naturally in many foods. The amount of selenium in plant foods depends on the amount of selenium in the soil where they were grown. The amount of selenium in animal products depends on the selenium content of the foods that the animals ate. You can get recommended amounts of selenium by eating a variety of foods, including the following:

- Seafood
- Meat, poultry, eggs, and dairy products
- Breads, cereals, and other grain products

What Kinds Of Selenium Dietary Supplements Are Available?

Selenium is available in many multivitamin-mineral supplements and other dietary supplements. It can be present in several different forms, including selenomethionine and sodium selenate.

Am I Getting Enough Selenium?

Most Americans get enough selenium from their diet because they eat food grown or raised in many different areas, including areas with soil that is rich in selenium.

Certain groups of people are more likely than others to have trouble getting enough selenium:

- People undergoing kidney dialysis

- People living with HIV

- People who eat only local foods grown in soils that are low in selenium

What Happens If I Don't Get Enough Selenium?

Selenium deficiency is very rare in the United States and Canada. Selenium deficiency can cause Keshan disease (a type of heart disease) and male infertility. It might also cause Kashin-Beck disease, a type of arthritis that produces pain, swelling, and loss of motion in your joints.

What Are Some Effects Of Selenium On Health?

Scientists are studying selenium to understand how it affects health. Here are some examples of what this research has shown.

Cancer

Studies suggest that people who consume lower amounts of selenium could have an increased risk of developing cancers of the colon and rectum, prostate, lung, bladder, skin, esophagus, and stomach. But whether selenium supplements reduce cancer risk is not clear. More research is needed to understand the effects of selenium from food and dietary supplements on cancer risk.

Cardiovascular Disease

Scientists are studying whether selenium helps reduce the risk of cardiovascular disease. Some studies show that people with lower blood levels of selenium have a higher risk of heart disease, but other studies do not. More studies are needed to better understand how selenium in food and dietary supplements affects heart health.

Cognitive Decline

Blood selenium levels decrease as people age, and scientists are studying whether low selenium levels contribute to a decline in brain function in the elderly. Some studies suggest that people with lower blood selenium levels are more likely to have poorer mental function. But a study of elderly people in the United States found no link between selenium levels and memory. More research is needed to find out whether selenium dietary supplements might help reduce the risk of or treat cognitive decline in elderly people.

Thyroid Disease

The thyroid gland has high amounts of selenium that play an important role in thyroid function. Studies suggest that people—especially women—who have low blood levels of selenium (and iodine) might develop problems with their thyroid. But whether selenium dietary supplements can help treat or reduce the risk of thyroid disease is not clear. More research is needed to understand the effects of selenium on thyroid disease.

Can Selenium Be Harmful?

Yes, if you get too much. Brazil nuts, for example, contain very high amounts of selenium (68–91 mcg per nut) and can cause you to go over the upper limit if you eat too many. Getting too much selenium over time can cause the following:

- Garlic breath
- Nausea
- Diarrhea
- Skin rashes
- Irritability
- Metallic taste in the mouth
- Brittle hair or nails
- Loss of hair or nails
- Discolored teeth
- Nervous system problems

Extremely high intakes of selenium can cause severe problems, including difficulty breathing, tremors, kidney failure, heart attacks, and heart failure.

The upper limit for selenium from foods and dietary supplements is listed below.

Table 22.5. Upper Limit For Selenium From Foods And Dietary Supplements

Ages	Upper Limit
Teens 14–18 years	400 mcg

Chapter 23

Multivitamin And Mineral (MVM) Dietary Supplements

What Are Multivitamin/Mineral (MVM) Dietary Supplements?

Multivitamin/mineral (MVM) supplements contain a combination of vitamins and minerals, and sometimes other ingredients as well. They go by many names, including *multis* and *multiples* or simply *vitamins*. The vitamins and minerals in MVMs have unique roles in the body.

What Kinds Of MVM Supplements Are Available?

There are many types of MVMs in the marketplace. Manufacturers choose which vitamins, minerals, and other ingredients, as well as their amounts, to include in their products.

Among the most common MVMs are basic, once-daily products containing all or most vitamins and minerals, with the majority in amounts that are close to recommended amounts. Higher-potency MVMs often come in packs of two or more pills to take each day. Manufacturers promote other MVMs for special purposes, such as better performance or energy, weight control, or improved immunity. These products usually contain herbal and other ingredients (such as echinacea and glucosamine) in addition to vitamins and minerals.

The recommended amounts of nutrients people should get vary by age and gender and are known as Recommended Dietary Allowances (RDAs) and Adequate Intakes (AIs). One value for each nutrient, known as the Daily Value (DV), is selected for the labels of dietary

About This Chapter: Information in this chapter is excerpted from "Multivitamin/Mineral Supplements," Office of Dietary Supplements (ODS), National Institutes of Health (NIH) February 17, 2016.

supplements and foods. A DV is often, but not always, similar to one's RDA or AI for that nutrient. The label provides the %DV so that you can see how much (what percentage) a serving of the product contributes to reaching the DV.

Who Takes MVM Supplements?

Research has shown that more than one-third of Americans take MVMs. About one in four young children takes an MVM, but adolescents are least likely to take them. Use increases with age during adulthood so that by age 71 years, more than 40% take an MVM.

Women; the elderly; people with more education, more income, healthier diets and lifestyles, and lower body weights; and people in the western United States use MVMs most often. Smokers and members of certain ethnic and racial groups (such as African Americans, Hispanics, and Native Americans) are less likely to take a daily MVM.

What Are Some Effects Of MVMs On Health?

People take MVMs for many reasons. Here are some examples of what research has shown about using them to increase nutrient intakes, promote health, and reduce the risk of disease.

Increase Nutrient Intakes

Taking an MVM increases nutrient intakes and helps people get the recommended amounts of vitamins and minerals when they cannot or do not meet these needs from food alone. But taking an MVM can also raise the chances of getting too much of some nutrients, like iron, vitamin A, zinc, niacin, and folic acid, especially when a person uses more than a basic, once-daily product.

Some people take an MVM as a form of dietary or nutritional "insurance." Ironically, people who take MVMs tend to consume more vitamins and minerals from food than those who don't. Also, the people least likely to get enough nutrients from diet alone who might benefit from MVMs are the least likely to take them.

Health Promotion And Chronic Disease Prevention

For people with certain health problems, specific MVMs might be helpful. For example, a study showed that a particular high-dose formula of several vitamins and minerals slowed vision loss in some people with age-related macular degeneration. Although a few studies show that MVMs might reduce the overall risk of cancer in certain men, most research shows that healthy people who take an MVM do not have a lower chance of getting cancer, heart disease, or diabetes. Based on current research, it's not possible to recommend for or against the use of MVMs to stay healthier longer.

One reason we know so little about whether MVMs have health benefits is that studies often use different products, making it hard to compare their results to find patterns. Many MVMs are available, and manufacturers can change their composition at will. It is therefore difficult for researchers to study whether a specific combination of vitamins and minerals affects health. Also, people with healthier diets and lifestyles are more likely to take dietary supplements, making it hard to identify any benefits from the MVMs.

Should I Take An MVM?

MVMs cannot take the place of eating a variety of foods that are important to a healthy diet. Foods provide more than vitamins and minerals. They also have fiber and other ingredients that may have positive health effects. But people who don't get enough vitamins and minerals from food alone, are on low-calorie diets, have a poor appetite, or avoid certain foods (such as strict vegetarians and vegans) might consider taking an MVM. Healthcare providers might also recommend MVMs to patients with certain medical problems.

Some people might benefit from taking certain nutrients found in MVMs. For example:

- Women who might become pregnant should get 400 mcg/day of folic acid from fortified foods and/or dietary supplements to reduce the risk of birth defects of the brain and spine in their newborn babies.

- Pregnant women should take an iron supplement as recommended by their healthcare provider. A prenatal MVM is likely to provide iron.

- Breastfed and partially breastfed infants should receive vitamin D supplements of 400 IU/day, as should non-breastfed infants who drink less than about 1 quart per day of vitamin D-fortified formula or milk.

- In postmenopausal women, calcium and vitamin D supplements may increase bone strength and reduce the risk of fractures.

- People over age 50 should get recommended amounts of vitamin B12 from fortified foods and/or dietary supplements because they might not absorb enough of the B12 that is naturally found in food.

Can MVMs Be Harmful?

Taking a basic MVM is unlikely to pose any risks to health. But if you consume fortified foods and drinks (such as cereals or beverages with added vitamins and minerals) or take other dietary supplements, make sure that the MVM you take doesn't cause your intake of any vitamin or mineral to go above the upper levels.

Pay particular attention to the amounts of vitamin A, beta-carotene (which the body can convert to vitamin A), and iron in the MVM.

- Women who get too much vitamin A during pregnancy can increase the risk of birth defects in their babies. This risk does not apply to beta-carotene, however. Smokers, and perhaps former smokers, should avoid MVMs with large amounts of beta-carotene and vitamin A because these ingredients might increase the risk of developing lung cancer.

- When the body takes in much more iron than it can eliminate, the iron can collect in body tissues and organs, such as the liver and heart, and damage them. Iron supplements are a leading cause of poisoning in children under age 6, so keep any products containing iron (such as children's chewable MVMs or adults' iron supplements) out of children's reach.

Chapter 24

What You Need To Know About Dietary Supplements

You've heard about them, may have used them, and may have even recommended them to friends or family. While some dietary supplements are well understood and established, others need further study. Read on for important information for you and your family about dietary supplements.

Before making decisions about whether to take a supplement, talk to your healthcare provider. They can help you achieve a balance between the foods and nutrients you personally need.

What Are Dietary Supplements?

Dietary supplements include such ingredients as vitamins, minerals, herbs, amino acids, and enzymes. Dietary supplements are marketed in forms such as tablets, capsules, softgels, gelcaps, powders, and liquids.

What Are The Benefits Of Dietary Supplements?

Some supplements can help assure that you get enough of the vital substances the body needs to function; others may help reduce the risk of disease. But supplements should not replace complete meals which are necessary for a healthful diet—so, be sure you eat a variety of foods as well.

About This Chapter: Information in this chapter is excerpted from "Dietary Supplements: What You Need to Know," U.S. Food and Drug Administration (FDA), January 6, 2016; and information from "Questions and Answers on Dietary Supplements," U.S. Food and Drug Administration (FDA), January 13, 2016.

Unlike drugs, **supplements are not intended to treat, diagnose, prevent, or cure diseases**. That means supplements should not make claims, such as "reduces pain" or "treats heart disease." Claims like these can only legitimately be made for drugs, not dietary supplements.

Are There Any Risks In Taking Supplements?

Yes. Many supplements contain active ingredients that have strong biological effects in the body. This could make them unsafe in some situations and hurt or complicate your health. For example, the following actions could lead to harmful—even life-threatening—consequences.

- combining supplements

- using supplements with medicines (whether prescription or over-the-counter)

- substituting supplements for prescription medicines

- taking too much of some supplements, such as vitamin A, vitamin D, or iron

- some supplements can also have unwanted effects *before, during, and after* surgery. So, be sure to inform your healthcare provider, including your pharmacist about any supplements you are taking

Some Common Dietary Supplements

- Calcium
- Chondroitin Sulphate
- Echinacea
- Fish Oil
- Garlic
- Ginkgo

- Ginseng
- Glucosamine
- Green Tea
- Saw Palmetto
- St. John's Wort
- Vitamin D

How Can I Find Out More About The Dietary Supplement I'm Taking?

Dietary supplement labels must include name and location information for the manufacturer or distributor.

If you want to know more about the product that you are taking, check with the manufacturer or distributor about:

- Information to support the claims of the product

- Information on the safety and effectiveness of the ingredients in the product.

How Can I Be A Smart Supplement Shopper?

Be a savvy supplement user. Here's how:

- When searching for supplements on the internet, use noncommercial sites (e.g., NIH, FDA, USDA) rather than doing blind searches.

- Watch out for false statements like "works better than [a prescription drug]," "totally safe," or has "no side effects."

- Be aware that the term *natural* doesn't always means *safe*.

- Ask your healthcare provider for help in distinguishing between reliable and questionable information.

- Always remember–safety first!

What Is A Dietary Supplement?

Congress defined the term "dietary supplement" in the Dietary Supplement Health and Education Act (DSHEA) of 1994. A dietary supplement is a product taken by mouth that contains a "dietary ingredient" intended to supplement the diet. The "dietary ingredients" in these products may include: vitamins, minerals, herbs or other botanicals, amino acids, and substances such as enzymes, organ tissues, glandulars, and metabolites. Dietary supplements can also be extracts or concentrates, and may be found in many forms such as tablets, capsules, softgels, gelcaps, liquids, or powders. They can also be in other forms, such as a bar, but if they are, information on their label must not represent the product as a conventional food or a sole item of a meal or diet. Whatever their form may be, DSHEA places dietary supplements in a special category under the general umbrella of "foods," not drugs, and requires that every supplement be labeled a dietary supplement.

What Is A "New Dietary Ingredient" In A Dietary Supplement?

The Dietary Supplement Health and Education Act (DSHEA) of 1994 defined both of the terms "dietary ingredient" and "new dietary ingredient" as components of dietary supplements.

In order for an ingredient of a dietary supplement to be a "dietary ingredient," it must be one or any combination of the following substances:

- a vitamin,

- a mineral,

- an herb or other botanical,

- an amino acid,

- a dietary substance for use by man to supplement the diet by increasing the total dietary intake (e.g., enzymes or tissues from organs or glands), or

- a concentrate, metabolite, constituent or extract.

A "new dietary ingredient" is one that meets the above definition for a "dietary ingredient" and was not sold in the United States in a dietary supplement before October 15, 1994.

What Information Must The Manufacturer Disclose On The Label Of A Dietary Supplement?

U.S. Food and Drug Administration (FDA) regulations require that certain information appear on dietary supplement labels. Information that must be on a dietary supplement label includes: a descriptive name of the product stating that it is a "supplement"; the name and place of business of the manufacturer, packer, or distributor; a complete list of ingredients; and the net contents of the product. In addition, each dietary supplement (except for some small volume products or those produced by eligible small businesses) must have nutrition labeling in the form of a "Supplement Facts" panel. This label must identify each dietary ingredient contained in the product.

Must All Ingredients Be Declared On The Label Of A Dietary Supplement?

Yes, ingredients not listed on the "Supplement Facts" panel must be listed in the "other ingredient" statement beneath the panel. The types of ingredients listed there could include the source of dietary ingredients, if not identified in the "Supplement Facts" panel (e.g., rose hips as the source of vitamin C), other food ingredients (e.g., water and sugar), and technical additives or processing aids (e.g., gelatin, starch, colors, stabilizers, preservatives, and flavors).

Is It Legal To Market A Dietary Supplement Product As A Treatment Or Cure For A Specific Disease Or Condition?

No, a product sold as a dietary supplement and promoted on its label or in labeling* as a treatment, prevention or cure for a specific disease or condition would be considered an unapproved—and thus illegal—drug. To maintain the product's status as a dietary supplement, the label and labeling must be consistent with the provisions in the Dietary Supplement Health and Education Act (DSHEA) of 1994.

Labeling refers to the label as well as accompanying material that is used by a manufacturer to promote and market a specific product.

Why Do Some Supplements Have Wording (A Disclaimer) That Says: "This Statement Has Not Been Evaluated By The FDA. This Product Is Not Intended To Diagnose, Treat, Cure, Or Prevent Any Disease"?

This statement or "disclaimer" is required by law (DSHEA) when a manufacturer makes a structure/function claim on a dietary supplement label. In general, these claims describe the role of a nutrient or dietary ingredient intended to affect the structure or function of the body. The manufacturer is responsible for ensuring the accuracy and truthfulness of these claims; they are not approved by FDA. For this reason, the law says that if a dietary supplement label includes such a claim, it must state in a "disclaimer" that FDA has not evaluated this claim. The disclaimer must also state that this product is not intended to "diagnose, treat, cure or prevent any disease," because only a drug can legally make such a claim.

How Do I, My Healthcare Provider, Or Any Informed Individual Report A Problem Or Illness Caused By A Dietary Supplement To FDA?

If you think you have suffered a serious harmful effect or illness from a dietary supplement, the first thing you should do is contact or see your healthcare provider immediately. Then, you or your healthcare provider can report this by submitting a report through the Safety

Reporting Portal. If you do not have access to the internet, you may submit a report by calling FDA's MedWatch hotline at 1-800-332-1088 (1-800-FDA-1088).

Report Problems To FDA

Notify FDA if the use of a dietary supplement caused you or a family member to have a serious reaction or illness (even if you are not certain that the product was the cause or you did not visit a doctor or clinic).

Follow these steps:

1. Stop using the product.

2. Contact your healthcare provider to find out how to take care of the problem.

3. Report problems to FDA in either of these ways:

    • Contact the Consumer Complaint Coordinator in your area

    • File a safety report online through the Safety Reporting Portal

Part Three
Other Elements Inside Food

Chapter 25
Sodium: Salt By Any Name

Is It Salt Or Sodium?

Sodium chloride is the chemical name for dietary salt. The words "salt" and "sodium" are not exactly the same, but consumers often use them interchangeably. The use of both terms may be seen on food packaging; for example, the Nutrition Facts label uses "sodium," whereas the front of the package may say "salt free." Ninety percent of the sodium we consume is in the form of salt.

Why Is Reducing Sodium Intake Important?

High sodium intake raises blood pressure, and high blood pressure is a major cause of heart disease and stroke. Even if a person does not have high blood pressure, reducing sodium intake is important because the lower one's blood pressure in general, the lower the risk for heart disease and stroke. The average daily sodium intake for Americans aged 2 years and older is more than 3,400 milligrams (mg). For American adults, the recommendation is to consume less than 2,300 mg of sodium each day. Reducing average population sodium consumption by 400 mg has been projected to prevent up to 28,000 deaths from any cause and save $7 billion in healthcare expenditures annually.

What Are The Dietary Guidelines For Sodium?

The *2015–2020 Dietary Guidelines for Americans* recommend Americans consume less than 2,300 mg of sodium each day as part of a healthy eating pattern.

About This Chapter: Information in this chapter is excerpted from "Sodium: Q and A," Centers for Disease Control and Prevention (CDC), April 2016; and information from "Labeling and Nutrition," U.S. Food and Drug Administration (FDA), June 2, 2016.

Where Does Most Of The Sodium In Our Diet Come From?

Most of the sodium we eat comes from processed foods and foods prepared in restaurants. When sodium is added to processed foods, it cannot be removed. More than 40 percent of sodium intake comes from the following of foods:

- Breads and rolls

- Cheese

- Cold cuts and cured meats such as deli or packaged ham or turkey

- Fresh and processed poultry

- Meat-mixed dishes such as meat loaf with tomato sauce

- Pasta dishes (not including macaroni and cheese)

- Pizza

- Sandwiches such as cheeseburgers

- Snacks such as chips, pretzels, and popcorn

- Soups

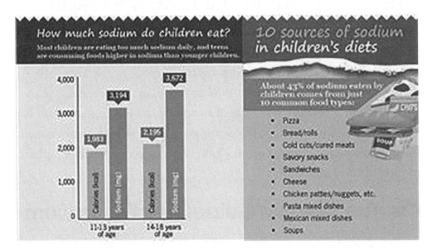

Figure 25.1. Sodium In Children's Diet

Source: "Reducing Sodium in Children's Diets," Vital Signs, Centers for Disease Control and Prevention (CDC), September 2014.

But remember, the sodium content can vary significantly between similar types of foods. So, use the Nutrition Facts Label to compare the amount of sodium in different foods and beverages, and select products that are lower in sodium. And, don't forget to check the serving size when comparing products in order to make an accurate comparison.

Can't Individuals Reduce Their Sodium Intake On Their Own?

Although some foods are high in sodium, excess sodium intake also is from frequent consumption of foods with only moderate amounts of sodium, such as breads and poultry. Additionally, different brands of the same foods may have different sodium levels. For example, sodium in chicken noodle soup can vary by as much as 840 mg per serving. Americans also eat outside the home frequently, and many restaurant foods do not have nutrition labels, so consumers often underestimate the amount of sodium, calories, and fat in restaurant meals. For all of these reasons, lowering personal sodium intake can be difficult. Gradually lowering the sodium content of the entire food supply will create greater choice for consumers who want or need to reduce sodium intake.

What Does "Salt Sensitive" Mean? Who Is "Salt Sensitive"?

Although nearly everyone can benefit from sodium reduction, some people are more salt sensitive than others—that is, they experience greater changes in blood pressure in relation to changes in sodium consumption. These individuals often include those who are older, black, have high blood pressure, have diabetes, or have chronic kidney disease. Currently, no screening test exists for salt sensitive people.

Table Salt Provides Iodine. Will Reducing Salt Intake Lead To Iodine Deficiency?

The majority of the sodium Americans consume comes from processed and restaurant foods. In the United States, salt used in food processing is not iodized. Reducing sodium in these foods would have minimal impact on iodine status in the population.

How Will Reducing Sodium Affect The Taste Of Foods?

Research has found that sodium reductions of up to 20 percent are not noticeable to consumers, depending on the food product. Consuming less sodium may decrease a person's preference for salt or sodium and lead to reduced consumption.

What Can Individuals Do To Lower Sodium Consumption?

- Choose to purchase healthy options and talk with your grocer or favorite restaurant about stocking lower sodium food choices.

- Read the Nutrition Facts label while shopping to find the lowest sodium options of your favorite foods. Foods considered low in sodium have less than 5 percent of the daily value of sodium.

- Eat a diet rich in fresh fruits and vegetables, frozen fruits and vegetables without sauce, and no salt added canned vegetables.

- Limit processed foods high in sodium.

- When eating out, request lower sodium options.

- Support initiatives that reduce sodium in foods in cafeterias and vending machines.

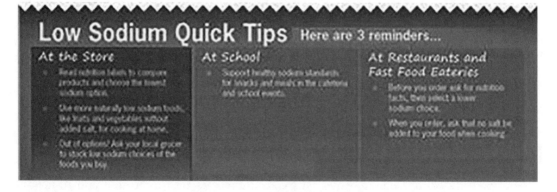

Figure 25.2. Low Sodium Quick Tips

Source: "Reducing Sodium in Children's Diets," Vital Signs, Centers for Disease Control and Prevention (CDC), September 2014.

Look At The Label!

Packaged foods and beverages can contain high levels of sodium, whether or not they **taste** salty. That's why it's important to use the Nutrition Facts Label to check the sodium content.

- **Understand the Daily Value.** The Daily Values are the amounts of nutrients recommended per day for Americans 4 years of age and older. The Daily Value for sodium is **less than 2,400 milligrams (mg) per day.**

- **Use the Percent Daily Value (%DV) as a tool.** The %DV tells you how much of a nutrient is in **one serving** of a food. The %DV is based on 100% of the Daily Value for sodium. When comparing and choosing foods, pick the food with a lower %DV of sodium. As a general rule:

  - 5% DV or less of sodium per serving is low

  - 20% DV or more of sodium per serving is high

- **Pay attention to serving sizes.** The %DV listed is for **one serving**, but one package may contain more than one serving. Be sure to look at the serving size to determine how many servings you are actually consuming. For example, if a package contains **two servings** and you eat the entire package, you are consuming **twice the amount** of sodium listed on the label.

Sodium As A Food Ingredient

As a food ingredient, sodium has multiple uses, such as for curing meat, baking, thickening, retaining moisture, enhancing flavor (including the flavor of other ingredients), and as a preservative. Some common food additives–like monosodium glutamate (MSG), sodium bicarbonate (baking soda), sodium nitrite, and sodium benzoate–also contain sodium and contribute (in lesser amounts) to the total amount of "sodium" listed on the Nutrition Facts Label.

Surprisingly, some foods that don't taste salty can still be high in sodium, which is why using taste alone is not an accurate way to judge a food's sodium content. For example, while some foods that are high in sodium (like pickles and soy sauce) **taste** salty, there are also many foods (like cereals and pastries) that contain sodium but **don't** taste salty. Also, some foods that you may eat several times a day (such as breads) can add up to a lot of sodium over the course of a day, even though an individual serving may not be high in sodium.

Check The Package For Nutrient Claims

You can also check for nutrient claims on food and beverage packages to quickly identify those that may contain less sodium. Here's a guide to common claims and what they mean:

Table 25.1. Package For Nutrient Claims

What It Says	What It Means
Salt/Sodium-Free	Less than 5 mg of sodium per serving
Very Low Sodium	35 mg of sodium or less per serving
Low Sodium	140 mg of sodium or less per serving
Reduced Sodium	At least 25% less sodium than the regular product
Light in Sodium or Lightly Salted	At least 50% less sodium than the regular product
No-Salt-Added or Unsalted	No salt is added during processing – but these products may not be salt/sodium-free unless stated

Sodium And Blood Pressure

Sodium attracts water, and a high-sodium diet draws water into the bloodstream, which can increase the volume of blood and subsequently your blood pressure. **High blood pressure** (also known as **hypertension**) is a condition in which blood pressure remains elevated over time. Hypertension makes the heart work harder, and the high force of the blood flow can harm arteries and organs (such as the heart, kidneys, brain, and eyes).

And since blood pressure normally rises with age, limiting your sodium intake becomes even more important each year. The good news is that eating less sodium can help lower blood pressure, which in turn, can help reduce your risk of developing these serious medical conditions.

Health Facts

Approximately 10 percent of children in the United States (ages 8 to 17 years old) have either hypertension or prehypertension.

Americans eat on average over **3,400 mg of sodium per day**, with intakes generally higher for men than women. However, the *Dietary Guidelines for Americans* recommends that adults and children ages 14 years and older limit sodium intake to **less than 2,300 mg per day**–that's equal to about **1 teaspoon of salt!**

10 Easy Tips For Reducing Sodium Consumption

Learning about sodium in foods and exploring new ways to prepare foods can help you achieve your sodium goal. And, if you follow these tips to reduce the amount of sodium you consume, your "taste" for sodium will gradually decrease over time—so eventually, you may not even miss it!

1. **Read the Nutrition Facts Label**

   Read the Nutrition Facts Label to see how much sodium is in foods and beverages. Most people should consume less than 100 percent of the Daily Value (or less than 2,400 mg) of sodium each day. Check the label to compare sodium in different brands of foods and beverages and choose those lower in sodium.

2. **Prepare your own food when you can**

   Limit packaged sauces, mixes, and "instant" products (including flavored rice, instant noodles, and ready-made pasta).

3. **Add flavor without adding sodium**

   Limit the amount of salt you add to foods when cooking, baking, or at the table. Try no-salt seasoning blends and herbs and spices instead of salt to add flavor to your food.

4. **Buy fresh**

   Choose fresh meat, poultry, and seafood, rather than processed varieties. Also, check the package on fresh meat and poultry to see if salt water or saline has been added.

5. **Watch your veggies**

   Buy fresh, frozen (no sauce or seasoning), or low sodium or no-salt-added canned vegetables.

6. **Give sodium the "rinse"**

   Rinse sodium-containing canned foods, such as beans, tuna, and vegetables before eating. This removes some of the sodium.

7. **"Unsalt" your snacks**

   Choose low sodium or no-salt-added nuts, seeds, and snack products (such as chips and pretzels)—or have carrot or celery sticks instead.

8. **Consider your condiments**

   Sodium in condiments can add up. Choose light or reduced sodium condiments, add oil and vinegar to salads rather than bottled dressings, and use only a small amount of seasoning from flavoring packets instead of the entire packet.

9. **Reduce your portion size**

   Less food means less sodium. Prepare smaller portions at home and consume less when eating out—choose smaller sizes, split an entrée with a friend, or take home part of your meal.

10. **Make lower-sodium choices at restaurants**

    Ask for your meal to be prepared without salt and request that sauces and salad dressings be served "on the side," then use less of them. If a restaurant item or meal includes a claim about its nutrient content, such as "low sodium" or "low fat," then nutrition information to support that claim is required to be available at the point of purchase.

Chapter 26
Carbohydrates

Carbohydrates are the body's main source of energy. They are sometimes called "carbs" for short. If you have heard of low-carb diets, you may think carbs are bad for you. Well, eating some carbohydrates is important. They help your body store energy for later use. Keep reading to learn more about:

- Types of carbohydrates
- Choosing carbohydrates

Types Of Carbohydrates

The carbohydrate group includes simple carbohydrates, complex carbohydrates, and fiber.

Simple carbohydrates are "simple" because they are in the most basic form. They are also sometimes called simple sugars. They include the sugar in sugar bowls and in candy. They also include the kinds of sugar that are naturally in fruits, vegetables, and milk. So, if fruit and candy both have sugar, why should you pick the fruit? Fruit has lots of other nutrients that are great for your health. An orange, for example, has vitamin C that is good for your skin.

Complex carbohydrates are "complex" because they are made of lots of simple sugars strung together. They are also called starches. They include bread, cereal, and pasta. They also include certain vegetables, like potatoes, peas, and corn. Your body needs to break starches down into sugars to use them for energy.

About This Chapter: Information in this chapter is excerpted from "Carbohydrates," Office on Women's Health (OWH), U.S. Department of Health and Human Services (HHS), November 5, 2013.

Fiber comes in many forms, like the outer parts of rice and other grains. Fiber offers a lot of health benefits, including helping with digestion. Also, because your body can't break it down, fiber helps you feel full. That means you may be less likely to overeat.

Choosing Carbohydrates

Sure, you may want to have some sweet treats from time to time. Overall, though, try to choose carbohydrates that offer the best boost for your health. Here's some useful info to help you choose:

When Eating Grains, Choose Mostly Whole Grains

Grains are foods like wheat, rice, oats, and cornmeal. There are two main types of grains: whole grains and refined grains.

- **Whole grains** are foods like whole wheat bread, brown rice, whole cornmeal, and oatmeal. They offer lots of nutrients that your body needs, like vitamins, minerals, and fiber.

  - At least half the grains you eat should be whole grains.

  - It's not hard to figure out whether a product has a lot of whole grain. Just check the ingredients list on the package and see if a whole grain is one of the first few items listed.

  - Keep in mind that "multigrain," "100 percent wheat," and brown-looking bread are not necessarily whole grain breads.

- **Refined grains** mean that the food company has removed some of the grain—and, along with it, some of the great nutrients. That's why your best bet is whole grain.

- **Enriched products** means some of the nutrients have been added back in. If you eat products with refined grains, try to eat ones that are enriched.

Try To Eat Foods With Dietary Fiber

Foods that contain good amounts of fiber include fruits, veggies, beans, nuts, seeds, and whole grains.

- The Nutrition Facts label on the back of food packages tells you how much fiber a product has. Aim to eat a total of around 25 grams of fiber per day.

Try To Avoid Foods With A Lot Of Added Sugar

- Foods with a lot of sugar can have many calories but not much nutrition.

- Eating a lot of calories can lead to being an unhealthy weight, which can cause health problems such as diabetes and heart disease.

- Aim to keep added sugars to less than 10 percent of your calories. If you eat around 2,000 calories a day, that means you want no more than 200 calories to come from added sugar. A can of regular soda might have around 150 calories from added sugar.

- Things that have a lot of added sugars include fruit drinks, energy or sports drinks, cakes, cookies, donuts, and ice cream.

- You can tell if a food or drink has added sugars by looking at the list of ingredients. The ingredients are listed from the greatest amount to the least amount. If a type of sugar comes early in the list, it means the product has a lot of sugar.

- Types of added sugars include:

  - Corn sweetener and corn syrup

  - Dextrose

  - Fructose and high-fructose corn syrup

  - Glucose

  - Honey

  - Maltose

  - Molasses

  - Sucrose

  - Sugar and brown sugar

  - Syrup and malt syrup

Chapter 27

Sugars / Syrups (Added Sugars)

What Are Added Sugars?

Added sugars are sugars and syrups that are added to foods or beverages when they are processed or prepared. This does not include naturally occurring sugars such as those in milk and fruits.

The major food and beverage sources of added sugars for Americans are:

- regular soft drinks, energy drinks, and sports drinks

- candy

- cakes

- cookies

- pies and cobblers

- sweet rolls, pastries, and donuts

- fruit drinks, such as fruitades and fruit punch

- dairy desserts, such as ice cream

> Almost half of the added sugars in our diets come from drinks—like sodas, fruit drinks, and other sweetened beverages.

About This Chapter: Information in this chapter is excerpted from "What Are Added Sugars?" ChooseMyPlate.gov, U.S. Department of Agriculture (USDA), August 16, 2016; and information from "Cut Down on Added Sugars," 2015–2020 Dietary Guidelines for Americans, Office of Disease Prevention and Health Promotion (ODPHP), U.S. Department of Health and Human Services (HHS), March 2016.

Reading the ingredient label on processed foods can help to identify added sugars. Names for added sugars on food labels include:

- Anhydrous dextrose
- Brown sugar
- Confectioner's powdered sugar
- Corn syrup
- Corn syrup solids
- Dextrose
- Fructose
- High-fructose corn syrup (HFCS)
- Honey
- Invert sugar
- Lactose
- Malt syrup
- Maltose
- Maple syrup
- Molasses
- Nectars (e.g., peach nectar, pear nectar)
- Pancake syrup
- Raw sugar
- Sucrose
- Sugar
- White granulated sugar

You may also see other names used for added sugars, but these are not recognized by the FDA as an ingredient name. These include cane juice, evaporated corn sweetener, crystal dextrose, glucose, liquid fructose, sugar cane juice, and fruit nectar.

> The average American gets 270 calories of added sugars each day. That's about 17 teaspoons of sugar!

Chapter 28

Sugar Substitutes (High-Intensity Sweeteners)

High-intensity sweeteners are commonly used as sugar substitutes or sugar alternatives because they are many times sweeter than sugar but contribute only a few to no calories when added to foods. High-intensity sweeteners, like all other ingredients added to food in the United States, must be safe for consumption.

What Are High-Intensity Sweeteners?

High-intensity sweeteners are ingredients used to sweeten and enhance the flavor of foods. Because high-intensity sweeteners are many times sweeter than table sugar (sucrose), smaller amounts of high-intensity sweeteners are needed to achieve the same level of sweetness as sugar in food. People may choose to use high-intensity sweeteners in place of sugar for a number of reasons, including that they do not contribute calories or only contribute a few calories to the diet. High-intensity sweeteners also generally will not raise blood sugar levels.

Which High-Intensity Sweeteners Are Permitted For Use In Food?

Six high-intensity sweeteners are FDA-approved as food additives in the United States:

- Acesulfame potassium (Ace-K)
- Advantame
- Aspartame

About This Chapter: Information in this chapter is excerpted from "High-Intensity Sweeteners," U.S. Food and Drug Administration (FDA), May 19, 2014.

- Neotame

- Saccharin

- Sucralose

In What Foods Are High-Intensity Sweeteners Typically Found?

High-intensity sweeteners are widely used in foods and beverages marketed as "sugar-free" or "diet," including baked goods, soft drinks, powdered drink mixes, candy, puddings, canned foods, jams and jellies, dairy products, and scores of other foods and beverages.

How Do I Know If High-Intensity Sweeteners Are Used In A Particular Food Product?

Consumers can identify the presence of high-intensity sweeteners by name in the ingredient list on food product labels.

Are High-Intensity Sweeteners Safe To Eat?

Based on the available scientific evidence, the agency has concluded that the high-intensity sweeteners approved by FDA are safe for the general population under certain conditions of use.

Are There Any High-Intensity Sweeteners That Should Be Avoided By Some People?

Consumers with phenylketonuria (PKU), a rare genetic disorder, have a difficult time metabolizing phenylalanine, a component of aspartame, and should avoid or restrict aspartame consumption. Sensitive consumers can avoid food products containing aspartame by looking at the label of such products, which must include a statement to inform phenylketonurics that the product contains phenylalanine.

How Much High-Intensity Sweetener Is Safe To Eat?

During premarket review, FDA established an acceptable daily intake (ADI) level for each of the five high-intensity sweeteners approved as food additives. An ADI is the amount of a substance that is considered safe to consume each day over the course of a person's lifetime. For each of these sweeteners, FDA determined that the estimated daily intake even for a high consumer of the substance would not exceed the ADI. Generally, an additive does not present safety concerns if the estimated daily intake is less than the ADI.

Chapter 29
Which Fats Are Which?

Saturated, Unsaturated, And *Trans* Fats

To reduce your risk for heart disease, cut back on saturated fat and *trans* fat by replacing some foods high in saturated fat with unsaturated fat or oils.

Saturated Fat

Imagine a building made of solid bricks. This building of bricks is similar to the tightly packed bonds that make "saturated" fat. The bonds are often solid at room temperature like butter or the fat inside or around meat. Saturated fats are most often found in animal products such as beef, pork, and chicken. Leaner animal products, such as chicken breast or pork loin, often have less saturated fat. Foods that contain more saturated fat are usually solid at room temperature and are sometimes called "solid" fat.

Unsaturated Fat

Now, imagine the links in a chain that bend, move, and flow. The chain links are similar to the loose bonds that make "unsaturated" fat fluid or liquid at room temperature like the oil on top of a salad dressing or in a can of tuna. Unsaturated fat typically comes from plant sources such as olives, nuts, or seeds–but unsaturated fat is also present in fish. Unsaturated fat are usually called oils. Unlike saturated fat, these oils contain mostly monounsaturated and polyunsaturated fat.

About This Chapter: Information in this chapter is excerpted from "Saturated, Unsaturated, and *Trans* Fats," ChooseMyPlate.gov, U.S. Department of Agriculture (USDA), January 7, 2016; and information from "Nutrients And Health Benefits," ChooseMyPlate.gov, U.S. Department of Agriculture (USDA), October 23, 2015.

A few food products such as coconut oil, palm oils, or whole milk remain as liquids at room temperature but are high in saturated fat.

Trans Fats

Trans fat can be made from vegetable oils through a process called hydrogenation. *Trans* fat is naturally found in small amounts in some animal products such as meat, whole milk, and milk products. Check the food label to find out if *trans* fat is in your food choices. *Trans* fat can often be found in many cakes, cookies, crackers, icings, margarines, and microwave popcorn.

Limit Saturated And *Trans* Fat

Eating more unsaturated fat than saturated and *trans* fats can reduce your risk of heart disease and improve "good" (HDL) cholesterol levels. Replace foods high in saturated and *trans* fat such as butter, whole milk, and baked goods with foods higher in unsaturated fat found in plants and fish, such as vegetable oils, avocado, and tuna fish.

Some Common Foods Containing Saturated Fat

- beef fat (tallow, suet)
- butter
- chicken fat
- coconut oil
- cream
- hydrogenated oils
- milk fat
- palm and palm kernel oils
- partially hydrogenated oils
- pork fat (lard)
- shortening
- stick margerine

Cut back on foods containing saturated fat including:

- desserts and baked goods, such as cakes, cookies, donuts, pastries, and croissants
- fried chicken and other chicken dishes with the skin

- fried potatoes (French fries)–if fried in a saturated fat or hydrogenated oil

- ice cream and other dairy desserts

- many cheeses and foods containing cheese, such as pizza

- regular ground beef and cuts of meat with visible fat

- sausages, hot dogs, bacon, and ribs

- whole milk and full-fat dairy foods

Eating peanuts and certain tree nuts (i.e., walnuts, almonds, and pistachios) may reduce the risk of heart disease when consumed as part of a diet that is nutritionally adequate and within calorie needs. Because nuts and seeds are high in calories, eat them in small portions and use them to replace other protein foods, like some meat or poultry, rather than adding them to what you already eat. In addition, choose unsalted nuts and seeds to help reduce sodium intakes.

Oils As Part Of A Healthy Eating Style

Oils provide essential fatty acids and vitamin E. They are found in different plants such as soybeans, olives, corn, sunflowers, and peanuts. Choosing unsaturated oils instead of saturated fat can help you maintain a healthy eating style. A few plant oils, including coconut and palm oil, are higher in saturated fat and should be eaten less often.

Choose foods higher in unsaturated fat and lower in saturated fat as part of your healthy eating style.

- Use oil-based dressings and spreads on foods instead of butter, stick margarine, or cream cheese.

- Drink fat-free (skim) or low-fat (1 percent) milk instead of reduced-fat (2 percent) or whole milk.

- Buy lean cuts of meat instead of fatty meats or choose these foods less often.

- Add low-fat cheese to homemade pizza, pasta, and mixed dishes.

- In recipes, use low-fat plain yogurt instead of cream or sour cream.

Chapter 30
Food Ingredients, Additives, And Colors

For centuries, ingredients have served useful functions in a variety of foods. Our ancestors used salt to preserve meats and fish, added herbs and spices to improve the flavor of foods, preserved fruit with sugar, and pickled cucumbers in a vinegar solution. Nowadays, consumers demand and enjoy a food supply that is flavorful, nutritious, safe, convenient, colorful and affordable. Food additives and advances in technology help make that possible.

There are thousands of ingredients used to make foods. The U.S. Food and Drug Administration (FDA) maintains a list of over 3000 ingredients in its data base "Everything Added to Food in the United States", many of which we use at home every day (e.g., sugar, baking soda, salt, vanilla, yeast, spices, and colors).

Still, some consumers have concerns about additives because they may see the long, unfamiliar names and think of them as complex chemical compounds. In fact, every food we eat—whether a just-picked strawberry or a homemade cookie—is made up of chemical compounds that determine flavor, color, texture and nutrient value. All food additives are carefully regulated by federal authorities and various international organizations to ensure that foods are safe to eat and are accurately labeled.

The purpose of this chapter is to provide helpful background information about food and color additives: what they are, why they are used in foods and how they are regulated for safe use.

About This Chapter: Information in this chapter is excerpted from "Overview of Food Ingredients, Additives, and Colors," U.S. Food and Drug Administration (FDA), December 2, 2014.

Why Are Food And Color Ingredients Added To Food?

Additives perform a variety of useful functions in foods that consumers often take for granted. Some additives could be eliminated if we were willing to grow our own food, harvest and grind it, spend many hours cooking and canning, or accept increased risks of food spoilage. But most consumers today rely on the many technological, aesthetic and convenient benefits that additives provide.

Following are some reasons why ingredients are added to foods:

1. **To Maintain Or Improve Safety and Freshness:** Preservatives slow product spoilage caused by mold, air, bacteria, fungi or yeast. In addition to maintaining the quality of the food, they help control contamination that can cause foodborne illness, including life-threatening botulism. One group of preservatives—antioxidants—prevents fats and oils and the foods containing them from becoming rancid or developing an off-flavor. They also prevent cut fresh fruits such as apples from turning brown when exposed to air.

2. **To Improve Or Maintain Nutritional Value:** Vitamins and minerals (and fiber) are added to many foods to make up for those lacking in a person's diet or lost in processing, or to enhance the nutritional quality of a food. Such fortification and enrichment has helped reduce malnutrition in the United States and worldwide. All products containing added nutrients must be appropriately labeled.

3. **Improve Taste, Texture, And Appearance:** Spices, natural and artificial flavors, and sweeteners are added to enhance the taste of food. Food colors maintain or improve appearance. Emulsifiers, stabilizers and thickeners give foods the texture and consistency consumers expect. Leavening agents allow baked goods to rise during baking. Some additives help control the acidity and alkalinity of foods, while other ingredients help maintain the taste and appeal of foods with reduced fat content.

What Is A Food Additive?

In its broadest sense, a food additive is any substance added to food. Legally, the term refers to "any substance the intended use of which results or may reasonably be expected to result—directly or indirectly—in its becoming a component or otherwise affecting the characteristics of any food." This definition includes any substance used in the production, processing, treatment, packaging, transportation or storage of food. The purpose of the legal definition, however, is to impose a premarket approval requirement. Therefore, this definition excludes ingredients whose use is generally recognized as safe (where government approval is not needed), those ingredients approved for use by FDA or the U.S. Department of Agriculture prior to the food additives provisions of law, and color additives and pesticides where other legal premarket approval requirements apply.

Direct food additives are those that are added to a food for a specific purpose in that food. For example, xanthan gum—used in salad dressings, chocolate milk, bakery fillings, puddings and other foods to add texture—is a direct additive. Most direct additives are identified on the ingredient label of foods.

Indirect food additives are those that become part of the food in trace amounts due to its packaging, storage or other handling. For instance, minute amounts of packaging substances may find their way into foods during storage. Food packaging manufacturers must prove to the U.S. Food and Drug Administration (FDA) that all materials coming in contact with food are safe before they are permitted for use in such a manner.

What Is A Color Additive?

A color additive is any dye, pigment or substance which when added or applied to a food, drug or cosmetic, or to the human body, is capable (alone or through reactions with other substances) of imparting color. FDA is responsible for regulating all color additives to ensure that foods containing color additives are safe to eat, contain only approved ingredients and are accurately labeled.

Color additives are used in foods for many reasons:

1. to offset color loss due to exposure to light, air, temperature extremes, moisture and storage conditions;

2. to correct natural variations in color;

3. to enhance colors that occur naturally; and

4. to provide color to colorless and "fun" foods.

Without color additives, colas wouldn't be brown, margarine wouldn't be yellow and mint ice cream wouldn't be green. Color additives are now recognized as an important part of practically all processed foods we eat.

FDA's permitted colors are classified as subject to certification or **exempt from certification,** both of which are subject to rigorous safety standards prior to their approval and listing for use in foods.

- **Certified colors** are synthetically produced (or human made) and used widely because they impart an intense, uniform color, are less expensive, and blend more easily to create a variety of hues. There are nine certified color additives approved for use in the United States (e.g., FD&C Yellow No. 6.). Certified food colors generally do not add undesirable flavors to foods.

- Colors that are **exempt from certification** include pigments derived from natural sources such as vegetables, minerals or animals. Nature derived color additives are typically more expensive than certified colors and may add unintended flavors to foods. Examples of exempt colors include annatto extract (yellow), dehydrated beets (bluish-red to brown), caramel (yellow to tan), beta-carotene (yellow to orange) and grape skin extract (red, green).

How Are Additives Approved For Use In Foods?

Nowadays, food and color additives are more strictly studied, regulated and monitored than at any other time in history. FDA has the primary legal responsibility for determining their safe use. To market a new food or color additive (or before using an additive already approved for one use in another manner not yet approved), a manufacturer or other sponsor must first petition FDA for its approval. These petitions must provide evidence that the substance is safe for the ways in which it will be used. As a result of recent legislation, since 1999, indirect additives have been approved via a premarket notification process requiring the same data as was previously required by petition.

When evaluating the safety of a substance and whether it should be approved, FDA considers:

1. the composition and properties of the substance

2. the amount that would typically be consumed

3. immediate and long-term health effects, and

4. various safety factors

The evaluation determines an appropriate level of use that includes a built-in safety margin-a factor that allows for uncertainty about the levels of consumption that are expected to be harmless. In other words, the levels of use that gain approval are much lower than what would be expected to have any adverse effect.

Because of inherent limitations of science, FDA can never be *absolutely* certain of the absence of any risk from the use of any substance. Therefore, FDA must determine-based on the best science available-if there is a *reasonable certainty of no harm* to consumers when an additive is used as proposed.

If an additive is approved, FDA issues regulations that may include the types of foods in which it can be used, the maximum amounts to be used, and how it should be identified on food labels. In 1999, procedures changed so that FDA now consults with USDA during the review process for ingredients that are proposed for use in meat and poultry products. Federal officials then monitor the extent of Americans' consumption of the new additive and results of any new research on its safety to ensure its use continues to be within safe limits.

If new evidence suggests that a product already in use may be unsafe, or if consumption levels have changed enough to require another look, federal authorities may prohibit its use or conduct further studies to determine if the use can still be considered safe.

Regulations known as Good Manufacturing Practices (GMP) limit the amount of food ingredients used in foods to the amount necessary to achieve the desired effect.

Table 30.1. Types Of Food Ingredients

Types Of Ingredients	What They Do	Examples Of Uses	Names Found On Product Labels
Preservatives	Prevent food spoilage from bacteria, molds, fungi, or yeast (antimicrobials); slow or prevent changes in color, flavor, or texture and delay rancidity (antioxidants); maintain freshness	Fruit sauces and jellies, beverages, baked goods, cured meats, oils and margarines, cereals, dressings, snack foods, fruits and vegetables	Ascorbic acid, citric acid, sodium benzoate, calcium propionate, sodium erythorbate, sodium nitrite, calcium sorbate, potassium sorbate, BHA, BHT, EDTA, tocopherols (Vitamin E)
Sweeteners	Add sweetness with or without the extra calories	Beverages, baked goods, confections, table-top sugar, substitutes, many processed foods	Sucrose (sugar), glucose, fructose, sorbitol, mannitol, corn syrup, high fructose corn syrup, saccharin, aspartame, sucralose, acesulfame potassium (acesulfame-K), neotame

Table 30.1. Continued

Types Of Ingredients	What They Do	Examples Of Uses	Names Found On Product Labels
Color Additives	Offset color loss due to exposure to light, air, temperature extremes, moisture and storage conditions; correct natural variations in color; enhance colors that occur naturally; provide color to colorless and "fun" foods	Many processed foods, (candies, snack foods margarine, cheese, soft drinks, jams/jellies, gelatins, pudding and pie fillings)	FD&C Blue Nos. 1 and 2, FD&C Green No. 3, FD&C Red Nos. 3 and 40, FD&C Yellow Nos. 5 and 6, Orange B, Citrus Red No. 2, annatto extract, beta-carotene, grape skin extract, cochineal extract or carmine, paprika oleoresin, caramel color, fruit and vegetable juices, saffron (Note: Exempt color additives are not required to be declared by name on labels but may be declared simply as colorings or color added)
Flavors And Spices	Add specific flavors (natural and synthetic)	Pudding and pie fillings, gelatin dessert mixes, cake mixes, salad dressings, candies, soft drinks, ice cream, BBQ sauce	Natural flavoring, artificial flavor, and spices
Flavor Enhancers	Enhance flavors already present in foods (without providing their own separate flavor)	Many processed foods	Monosodium glutamate (MSG), hydrolyzed soy protein, autolyzed yeast extract, disodium guanylate or inosinate

Table 30.1. Continued

Types Of Ingredients	What They Do	Examples Of Uses	Names Found On Product Labels
Fat Replacers (and components of formulations used to replace fats)	Provide expected texture and a creamy "mouth-feel" in reduced-fat foods	Baked goods, dressings, frozen desserts, confections, cake and dessert mixes, dairy products	Olestra, cellulose gel, carrageenan, polydextrose, modified food starch, micro particulated egg white protein, guar gum, xanthan gum, whey protein concentrate
Nutrients	Replace vitamins and minerals lost in processing (enrichment), add nutrients that may be lacking in the diet (fortification)	Flour, breads, cereals, rice, macaroni, margarine, salt, milk, fruit beverages, energy bars, instant breakfast drinks	Thiamine hydrochloride, riboflavin (Vitamin B2), niacin, niacinamide, folate or folic acid, beta carotene, potassium iodide, iron or ferrous sulfate, alpha tocopherols, ascorbic acid, Vitamin D, amino acids (L-tryptophan, L-lysine, L-leucine, L-methionine)
Emulsifiers	Allow smooth mixing of ingredients, prevent separation Keep emulsified products stable, reduce stickiness, control crystallization, keep ingredients dispersed, and to help products dissolve more easily	Salad dressings, peanut butter, chocolate, margarine, frozen desserts	Soy lecithin, mono- and diglycerides, egg yolks, polysorbates, sorbitan monostearate
Stabilizers And Thickeners, Binders, Texturizers	Produce uniform texture, improve "mouth-feel"	Frozen desserts, dairy products, cakes, pudding and gelatin mixes, dressings, jams and jellies, sauces	Gelatin, pectin, guar gum, carrageenan, xanthan gum, whey

Table 30.1. Continued

Types Of Ingredients	What They Do	Examples Of Uses	Names Found On Product Labels
pH Control Agents And Acidulants	Control acidity and alkalinity, prevent spoilage	Beverages, frozen desserts, chocolate, low acid canned foods, baking powder	Lactic acid, citric acid, ammonium hydroxide, sodium carbonate
Leavening Agents	Promote rising of baked goods	Breads and other baked goods	Baking soda, monocalcium phosphate, calcium carbonate
Anti-Caking Agents	Keep powdered foods free-flowing, prevent moisture absorption	Salt, baking powder, confectioner's sugar	Calcium silicate, iron ammonium citrate, silicon dioxide
Humectants	Retain moisture	Shredded coconut, marshmallows, soft candies, confections	Glycerin, sorbitol
Yeast Nutrients	Promote growth of yeast	Breads and other baked goods	Calcium sulfate, ammonium phosphate
Dough Strengtheners And Conditioners	Produce more stable dough	Breads and other baked goods	Ammonium sulfate, azodicarbonamide, L-cysteine
Firming Agents	Maintain crispness and firmness	Processed fruits and vegetables	Calcium chloride, calcium lactate
Enzyme Preparations	Modify proteins, polysaccharides and fats	Cheese, dairy products, meat	Enzymes, lactase, papain, rennet, chymosin
Gases	Serve as propellant, aerate, or create carbonation	Oil cooking spray, whipped cream, carbonated beverages	Carbon dioxide, nitrous oxide

Part Four
Smart Eating Plans

Chapter 31

MyPlate Nutrition Guide: Building A Healthy Plate

Before you eat, think about what goes on your plate or in your cup or bowl. Foods like vegetables, fruits, whole grains, low-fat dairy products, and lean protein foods contain the nutrients you need without too many calories. Try some of these options.

Make half your plate fruits and vegetables.

- Eat red, orange, and dark-green vegetables, such as tomatoes, sweet potatoes, and broccoli, in main and side dishes

- Eat fruit, vegetables, or unsalted nuts as snacks—they are nature's original fast foods

Switch to skim or 1 percent milk.

- They have the same amount of calcium and other essential nutrients as whole milk, but less fat and calories

- Try calcium-fortified soy products as an alternative to dairy foods

Make at least half your grains whole.

- Choose 100 percent whole-grain cereals, breads, crackers, rice, and pasta

- Check the ingredients list on food packages to find whole-grain foods

Vary your protein food choices.

- Twice a week, make seafood the protein on your plate

- Eat beans, which are a *natural* source of fiber and protein

- Keep meat and poultry portions small and lean

About This Chapter: Information in this chapter is excerpted from "Let's Eat for the Health of It," ChooseMyPlate. gov, U.S. Department of Agriculture (USDA), June 2011. Reviewed September 2016; and information from "MyPlate," ChooseMyPlate.gov, U.S. Department of Agriculture (USDA), January 7, 2016.

Cut Back On Foods High In Solid Fats, Added Sugars, And Salt

Many people eat foods with too much solid fats, added sugars, and salt (sodium). Added sugars and fats load foods with extra calories you don't need. Too much sodium may increase your blood pressure.

Choose foods and drinks with little or no added sugars.

- Drink water instead of sugary drinks. There are about 10 packets of sugar in a 12-ounce can of soda

- Select fruit for dessert. Eat sugary desserts less often

- Choose 100 percent fruit juice instead of fruit-flavored drinks

Look out for salt (sodium) in foods you buy—it all adds up.

- Compare sodium in foods like soup, bread, and frozen meals—and choose the foods with lower numbers

- Add spices or herbs to season food without adding salt

Eat fewer foods that are high in solid fats.

- Make major sources of saturated fats—such as cakes, cookies, ice cream, pizza, cheese, sausages, and hot dogs—occasional choices, not everyday foods

- Select lean cuts of meats or poultry and fat-free or low-fat milk, yogurt, and cheese

- Switch from solid fats to oils when preparing food

Table 31.1. Examples Of Solid Fats And Oils

Solid Fats	Oils
Beef, pork, and chicken fat	Canola oil
Butter, cream, and milk fat	Corn oil
Coconut, palm, and palm kernel oils	Cottonseed oil
Hydrogenated oil	Olive oil
Partially hydrogenated oil	Peanut oil
Shortening	Safflower oil
Stick margarine	Sunflower oil
	Tub (soft) margarine
	Vegetable oil

Eat The Right Amount Of Calories For You

Everyone has a personal calorie limit. Staying within yours can help you get to or maintain a healthy weight. People who are successful at managing their weight have found ways to keep track of how much they eat in a day, even if they don't count every calorie.

Enjoy your food, but eat less.

- Get your personal daily calorie limit at www.ChooseMyPlate.gov and keep that number in mind when deciding what to eat

- Think before you eat…is it worth the calories

- Avoid oversized portions

- Use a smaller plate, bowl, and glass

- Stop eating when you are satisfied, not full

Cook more often at home, where you are in control of what's in your food.

When eating out, choose lower calorie menu options.

- Check posted calorie amounts

- Choose dishes that include vegetables, fruits, and/or whole grains

- Order a smaller portion or share when eating out

Write down what you eat to keep track of how much you eat.

If you drink alcoholic beverages, do so sensibly—limit to 1 drink a day for women or to 2 drinks a day for men.

Be Physically Active Your Way

Pick activities that you like and start by doing what you can, at least 10 minutes at a time. Every bit adds up, and the health benefits increase as you spend more time being active.

MyPlate

MyPlate is a reminder to find your healthy eating style and build it throughout your lifetime. Everything you eat and drink matters. The right mix can help you be healthier now and in the future. This means:

- Focus on variety, amount, and nutrition

- Choose foods and beverages with less saturated fat, sodium, and added sugars

- Start with small changes to build healthier eating styles

- Support healthy eating for everyone

Eating healthy is a journey shaped by many factors, including our stage of life, situations, preferences, access to food, culture, traditions, and the personal decisions we make over time. All your food and beverage choices count. MyPlate offers ideas and tips to help you create a healthier eating style that meets your individual needs and improves your health.

Build A Healthy Eating Style

All Food And Beverage Choices Matter—Focus On Variety, Amount, And Nutrition

- Focus on making healthy food and beverage choices from all five food groups including fruits, vegetables, grains, protein foods, and dairy to get the nutrients you need.

- Eat the right amount of calories for you based on your age, sex, height, weight, and physical activity level.

- Building a healthier eating style can help you avoid overweight and obesity and reduce your risk of diseases such as heart disease, diabetes, and cancer.

Choose An Eating Style Low In Saturated Fat, Sodium, And Added Sugars

- Use Nutrition Facts labels and ingredient lists to find amounts of saturated fat, sodium, and added sugars in the foods and beverages you choose.

- Look for food and drink choices that are lower in saturated fat, sodium, and added sugar.

  - Eating fewer calories from foods high in saturated fat and added sugars can help you manage your calories and prevent overweight and obesity. Most of us eat too many foods that are high in saturated fat and added sugar.

  - Eating foods with less sodium can reduce your risk of high blood pressure.

Make Small Changes To Create A Healthier Eating Style

- Think of each change as a personal "win" on your path to living healthier. Each MyWin is a change you make to build your healthy eating style. Find little victories that fit into your lifestyle and celebrate as a MyWin!

- Start with a few of these small changes

- Make half your plate fruits and vegetables

- Focus on whole fruits

- Vary your veggies

- Make half your grains whole grains

- Move to low-fat and fat-free dairy

- Vary your protein routine

- Eat and drink the right amount for you

Support Healthy Eating For Everyone

- Create settings where healthy choices are available and affordable to you and others in your community.

- Individuals can help others in their journey to make healthy eating a part of their lives.

Chapter 32
Eating Well To Live Well

Know How Your Body Works

Think of food as energy to charge up your battery for the day. Throughout the day, you use energy from the battery to think and move, so you need to eat regularly to keep powered up. This is called "energy balance" because you need to balance food (energy you take in) with activity (energy you spend).

Eating Healthy and Being Physically Active May Help You
- Do better in school
- Have more energy for other fun times, like hanging out with your friends
- Make friends who share your interests in dance, sports, or other activities
- Tone up and strengthen your muscles
- Improve your mood

How Much Energy Does Your Body Need?

You may have heard of calories, which measure the amount of energy in a food. There is no "right" number of calories that works for everyone. The number of calories you need depends on whether you are a girl or a boy, how old you are, and how active you are (which may not be the same every day).

About this Chapter: Information in this chapter is excerpted from "Take Charge of Your Health: A Guide for Teens," National Institute of Diabetes and Digestive and Kidney Diseases (NIDDK), May 2012. Reviewed September 2016.

Should You Diet?

Dieting may not be wise. Many teens try to lose weight by eating very little, cutting out whole groups of foods (like "carbs"), skipping meals, and fasting. These methods can leave out important foods your body needs. In fact, **unhealthy dieting may make you gain more weight** because it often leads to a cycle of eating very little, then overeating or binge eating because you are hungry. This can also affect your emotions and how you grow.

Other weight-loss tactics like smoking, self-induced vomiting, or using diet pills or laxatives (medicines that help people have bowel movements) can also lead to health problems.

Charge Up With Healthy Eating

Healthy eating involves taking control of how much and what types of food you eat. This chapter has information to help you

- control your food portions

- charge your battery with high-energy foods

- avoid pizza, candy, and fast food

- stay powered up all day

Control Your Food Portions

A **portion** is the amount of one food you eat at one time. Many people eat larger portions than they need, especially when eating away from home. Ready-to-eat meals (from a restaurant, grocery store, or school event) may have larger portions than you need. Follow the tips below to control portions.

When Eating Away from Home

- Order something small. Try a half-portion or healthy appetizer, like hummus (chickpea spread) with whole-wheat pitas or grilled chicken. If you order a large meal, take half of it home or split it with someone else at the table.

- Limit the amount of fast food you eat. When you do get fast food, say "no thanks" to super-sized or value-sized options, like those that come with fries and soda.

- Choose salad with low-fat dressing, a sandwich with mustard instead of mayo, or other meals that have fruits, veggies, and whole grains.

- Choose grilled options, like chicken, or remove breading from fried items. Avoid meals that use the words creamy, breaded, battered, or buttered.

When Eating At Home

- Take one serving out of a package and eat it off a plate instead of eating straight out of a box or bag. "What do all these numbers mean?" explains where you can find serving sizes.

- Avoid eating in front of the TV or while you are busy with other activities. It is easy to lose track of how much you are eating if you eat while doing other things.

- Eat slowly so your brain can get the message that your stomach is full. Your brain needs about 20 minutes before it gets the message.

Charge Your Battery With High-Energy Foods

Eating healthy is not just about the amount of food you eat. You need to make sure you're eating the types of food that charge you up. Strive to eat meals that include fruits, vegetables, whole grains, low-fat protein, and dairy. More information is below, and you can check out the meal planning tool at the end of this guide.

Fruits And Vegetables

Make half of your plate fruits and vegetables. Dark green, red, and orange vegetables, in particular, have high levels of the nutrients you need, such as vitamin C, calcium, and fiber. Adding spinach or romaine lettuce and tomato to your sandwich is an easy way to get more veggies in your meal.

Grains

Choose whole grains, like whole-wheat bread, brown rice, and oatmeal.

Protein

Power up with lean meats, like turkey on a sandwich, or chicken, seafood, eggs, beans, nuts, tofu, and other protein-rich foods.

Dairy

Build strong bones with fat-free or low-fat milk products. If you cannot digest lactose (the sugar in milk that causes some people stomach pain), choose soy or rice milk and low-fat yogurt.

Avoid Pizza, Candy, And Fast Food

You don't have to stop eating these items, but eating less of them may help you maintain a healthy weight. Pizza, candy, fast food, and sodas have lots of added sugar, solid fats, and sodium. A healthy eating plan is low in these items.

Added Sugars

Many foods, especially fruits, are naturally sweet. Other foods, like cookies, snack cakes, and brownies, have added sugars to make them taste better. These sugars add calories but not nutrients.

Solid Fats

Fat is important. It helps your body grow and develop; it is a source of energy; and it even keeps your skin and hair healthy. But some fats are better for you than others.

Solid fats are fats that are solid at room temperature, like butter, stick margarine, shortening, and lard. These fats often contain saturated and *trans* fats, which are high in calories and not heart healthy. Take it easy on foods like cakes, cookies, pizza, and fries, which often have a lot of solid fat.

Sodium

Your body needs a small amount of sodium (mostly found in salt). But eating too much sodium can raise your blood pressure, which is unhealthy for your heart and your body in general.

Processed foods, like those that are canned, frozen, or packaged, often have a lot of sodium. Fresh foods do not, but often cost more. If you can afford to, eat fresh foods and prepare your own low-salt meals. If you use packaged foods, check the amount of sodium listed on the Nutrition Facts label. Rinse canned vegetables to remove excess salt.

Snack Smart

- Fresh apples, berries, or grapes
- A handful of walnuts or almonds
- Low-fat or fat-free yogurt
- String cheese
- Peanut butter on whole-wheat crackers

Try to eat fewer than 2,300 mg of sodium per day. This equals about one teaspoon and includes salt that is already in prepared food, as well as salt you add when cooking or eating your food.

Your doctor knows more about your specific needs, so don't be afraid to ask her or him how much sodium you should be eating.

Stay Charged Up All Day

Skipping meals can lead to weight gain. Follow these tips to maintain a healthy weight:

- **Eat breakfast every day.** It gets your body going. You can even grab something on the go, like a piece of fruit and a slice of whole-grain bread.
- **Pack your lunch on school days.** If you pack your lunch, you can control the portions and make sure your meal is healthy.
- **Eat healthy snacks, and try not to skip meals.**
- **Eat dinner with your family.** When you eat with your family, you are more likely to eat a healthy meal, and you can take the time to catch up with each other.
- **Be involved in grocery shopping and meal planning at home.** If you're involved, you can make sure meals are healthy and taste good.

Get Moving

Being physically active may help you control your weight, increase flexibility and balance, and improve your mood. You don't have to do boring exercise routines. You can be active through daily activities, like taking the stairs instead of the elevator or escalator.

This can help you to

- Be active every day
- Get outside
- Have fun with your friends
- Stay active indoors, too

Be Active Every Day

Physical activity should be part of your daily life, whether you play sports, take P.E. (physical education) or other exercise classes, or even get from place to place by walking or bicycling. You should be physically active for 60 minutes a day, but you don't have to do it all at once!

Have Fun With Your Friends

Being active can be more fun with friends or family members. You may also find that you make friends when you join active clubs or community activities. Teach each other new games or activities, and keep things interesting by choosing a different activity each day:

- Sports

- Active games

- Other actions that get you moving, like walking around the mall

Support your friends and challenge them to be healthy with you.

Get Outside

Many teens spend a lot of time indoors on **"screen time"**: watching TV, surfing the web, or playing video games. Too much screen time can lead you to have excess body fat or a higher weight. Instead, be active outdoors to burn calories and get extra vitamin D on a sunny day.

How To Cut Back Your Screen Time

- Tape your favorite shows and watch them later to keep from zoning out and flipping through channels.

- Replace after-school TV and video-game time with physical activities in your home, school, or community.

Choose Activities You Like

Being physically active does not mean you have to join a gym or do a team sport. You can walk or bicycle around your neighborhood or even turn up the music and dance. Try some of these ideas:

- Shoot baskets
- Ride your bike (wear a helmet)
- Run
- Skateboard
- Jump rope or use a hula hoop
- Have a dance party with friends
- Play volleyball or flag football
- Move with a video game that tracks your motion

- Gradually reduce the time you spend using your phone, computer, or TV. Challenge your friends or family members to join you, and see who can spend the least amount of time in front of a screen each week.

- Set up a text-free time with your friends—a length of time when you can be physically active together and agree not to send or respond to text messages.

- Turn off your cell phone before you go to bed.

Stay Active Indoors, Too

On cold or wet days, screen time is not the only option. Find ways to be active inside:

- Play indoor sports or active games in your building or home, at a local recreation center, or in your school gym.

- Dance to your favorite music by yourself or with friends.

- If you have a gaming system, choose active dance and sports games that track your movement.

Take Your Time

- **Make changes slowly.** Do not expect to change your eating or activity habits overnight. Changing too much too fast can hurt your chances of success.

- **Look at ways you can make your eating and physical activity habits healthier.** Use a food and activity journal for 4 or 5 days, and write down everything you eat, your activities, and your emotions. Review your journal to get a picture of your habits. Do you skip breakfast? Are you physically active most days of the week? Do you eat when you are stressed?

- **Know what's holding you back.** Are there unhealthy snack foods at home that are too tempting? Is the food at your cafeteria too high in fat and added sugars? Do you find it hard to resist drinking several sweetened sodas a day because your friends do it?

- **Set a few realistic goals for yourself.** First, try replacing a couple of the sodas you drink with unsweetened beverages. Once you are drinking less soda, try cutting out all soda. Then, set a few more goals, like drinking low-fat or fat-free milk, eating more fruits, or getting more physical activity each day.

- **Use the information in this booklet and the following resources to help you.** Stay positive and focused by remembering why you want to be healthier—to look, feel, move, and learn better. Accept setbacks—if you don't meet one of your eating or physical activity goals one day, do not give up. Just try again the next day.

- **Get a buddy at school or someone at home to support your new habits.** Ask a friend, sibling, parent, or guardian to help you make changes and stick with your new habits.

Make It Work For You

Being healthy sounds like a lot of work, right? It doesn't have to be. This chart will help you plan healthy meals and work healthy habits into your day. Put this on your fridge or in your school locker for quick reminders.

Pick An Item From Each Food Category To Plan A Healthy Meal

Table 32.1. Food Category To Plan A Healthy Meal

Fruits and Veggies	Grains	Protein	Dairy
1 banana or apple	1 serving of oatmeal or whole-grain cereal (size of your fist)	1 scrambled or hard-boiled egg	1 cup fat-free or low-fat milk (or substitute soy or rice milk)
1 handful fresh berries or raisins	2 DVD-sized whole-grain waffles or buckwheat pancakes	1 serving of peanut butter (size of a ping-pong ball)	6- to 8-ounce yogurt pack (also high in protein!)
1 serving romaine lettuce or spinach (size of your fist)	2 slices whole-wheat bread	1 handful of walnuts or almonds	1 serving low-fat cottage cheese (size of your fist)
1 handful baby carrots, strips of peppers, or celery sticks	1 whole-grain pita	1 serving of hummus (size of a ping-pong ball)	1 slice of Swiss or provolone cheese
1 cup tomato or vegetable juice	1 whole-wheat tortilla	1 serving of sliced, lean turkey or ham (size of the palm of your hand)	1 stick of string cheese
1 snack pack of fruit salad (in natural juices, not syrup)	1 serving of brown rice (total amount should fit in your cupped hands)	½ can of tuna with mustard or light mayo	1 handful shredded low-fat mozzarella cheese
1 serving of tomato-based pasta sauce with vegetables (fits in one cupped hand)	2 whole-grain taco shells	1 serving of black beans (size of your fist)	1 serving of low-fat sour cream (size of a ping-pong ball)

Table 32.1. Continued

Fruits and Veggies	Grains	Protein	Dairy
1 serving of steamed broccoli, green beans, or other veggie (fits in one cupped hand)	1 serving of whole-grain pasta (total amount should fit in your cupped hands)	1 serving lean beef, grilled chicken, tofu, or baked fish (size of the palm of your hand)	1 serving non-fat frozen yogurt (size of your fist)

Sample Meals

Breakfast: one banana, a slice of whole-grain bread with peanut butter, and milk

Lunch: a turkey sandwich with cheese, dark leafy lettuce, tomato, and red peppers on whole-wheat bread

Dinner: two whole-grain taco shells with chicken or black beans, low-fat cheese, and romaine lettuce

Make Healthy Habits Part Of Your Day

Eating healthy and being active can be difficult because you spend much of your day in school and eat meals that are prepared by others. Be a Health Champion by becoming more involved in your meals and school activities. Here's a checklist to help you work healthy habits into your day.

Be A Health Champion!

- Each night, pack a healthy lunch and snacks for the next day

- Go to bed at a regular time every night to recharge your body and mind. Be sure to turn off your phone, TV, and other devices when you go to bed

- Eat breakfast

- Walk or bike to school if you live nearby and can safely do so.

- Drink water throughout the day. Avoid sodas and other high-calorie drinks.

- Between classes, stand up and walk around, even if your next subject is in the same room.

- If a recess is allowed at your school, be sure to take a walk, jump rope, or play an active game with friends.

- Be active in gym classes.

- At lunchtime, eat the lunch you packed. If you have lunch money, spend it on healthy options. Avoid sodas, chips, and candy from the vending machines.

- Stay active after school by joining a sports team or dance group. Walk the dog or jump into a neighborhood pick-up game of basketball, soccer, or softball.

- Be involved in the food choices made in your home. Help make dinner and eat with your family.

- Save screen time for after your activities and limit it to less than 2 hours.

Chapter 33

Food Shopping Tips

Buying healthy foods for your family is easier when you know what types of food to shop for in the store. Take a shopping list with you to stay on track. Look at the Nutrition Facts label to find healthy choices.

Once you know how to use the Nutrition Facts label, be sure to read them as you shop. Look at the serving size and servings per container of the foods you may buy. Compare the total calories in similar products and choose the lowest calorie items.

Why The Nutrition Facts Label Is Important

- **Check servings and calories.** Look at the serving size and how many servings the package contains. If you eat one serving, the label clearly outlines the nutrients you get. If you eat two servings, you double the calories and nutrients, including the Percent Daily Value (% DV). The Daily Value is how much of a specific nutrient you need to eat in a day. Percent Daily Value tells you how much of a nutrient is in one serving of food compared to the amount you need each day.

- **Make your calories count.** Look at the calories on the label and note where the calories are coming from (fat, protein, or carbohydrates). Compare them with nutrients (like vitamins and minerals) to decide whether the food is a healthy choice.

- **Don't sugar-coat it.** Sugars add calories with few, if any, nutrients. Look for foods and beverages low in added sugars. Read the ingredient list and make sure that added sugars

About This Chapter: Information in this chapter is excerpted from "Food Shopping Tips," We Can!®, National Heart, Lung, and Blood Institute (NHLBI), February 13, 2013; and information from "Smart Shopping for Veggies and Fruits," ChooseMyPlate.gov, U.S. Department of Agriculture (USDA), September 2011. Reviewed September 2016.

are not one of the first few ingredients. Some names for added sugars include *sucrose, glucose, high-fructose corn syrup, corn syrup, maple syrup, and fructose.*

- **Know your fats.** Look for foods low in saturated fats, *trans* fats, and cholesterol to help reduce the risk of heart disease (5%DV or less is low, 20%DV or more is high). Keep total fat intake between 20% to 35% of calories.

- **Reduce sodium (salt), increase potassium.** Research shows that eating less than 2,300 milligrams of sodium (about one teaspoon of salt) per day might reduce the risk of high blood pressure. Most of the sodium people eat comes from processed foods, not from the salt shaker. Also, look for foods high in potassium (tomatoes, bananas, potatoes, and orange juice), which cancels out some of sodium's effects on blood pressure.

10 Tips For Affordable Vegetables And Fruits

1. Use fresh vegetables and fruits that are in season. They are easy to get, have more flavor, and are usually less expensive. Your local farmer's market is a great source of seasonal produce.

2. Check the local newspaper, online, and at the store for sales, coupons, and specials that will cut food costs. Often, you can get more for less by visiting larger grocery stores (discount grocers if available).

3. Plan out your meals ahead of time and make a grocery list. You will save money by buying only what you need. Don't shop when you're hungry. Shopping after eating will make it easier to pass on the tempting snack foods. You'll have more of your food budget for vegetables and fruits.

4. Compare the price and the number of servings from fresh, canned, and frozen forms of the same veggie or fruit. Canned and frozen items may be less expensive than fresh. For canned items, choose fruit canned in 100% fruit juice and vegetables with "low sodium" or "no salt added" on the label.

5. Some fresh vegetables and fruits don't last long. Buy small amounts more often to ensure you can eat the foods without throwing any away.

6. For fresh vegetables or fruits you use often, a large size bag is the better buy. Canned or frozen fruits or vegetables can be bought in large quantities when they are on sale, since they last much longer.

7. Opt for store brands when possible. You will get the same or similar product for a cheaper price. If your grocery store has a membership card, sign up for even more savings.

8. Buy vegetables and fruits in their simplest form. Pre-cut, pre-washed, ready-to-eat, and processed foods are convenient, but often cost much more than when purchased in their basic forms.

9. Start a garden—in the yard or a pot on the deck—for fresh, inexpensive, flavorful additions to meals. Herbs, cucumbers, peppers, or tomatoes are good options for beginners. Browse through a local library or online for more information on starting a garden.

10. Prepare and freeze vegetable soups, stews, or other dishes in advance. This saves time and money. Add leftover vegetables to casseroles or blend them to make soup. Overripe fruit is great for smoothies or baking.

Chapter 34
Eating Well While Eating Out

Why Does It Matter?

It's easy to be tempted when you're eating away from home—especially if everyone around you is chowing down on unhealthy options.

But eating too much fast food or always choosing high-fat, high-calorie menu items can drag a person's body down. The most obvious problem is weight gain. But because the food we eat affects how our bodies function, eating the right (or wrong) foods can influence any number of things:

- mental functioning
- emotional well-being
- energy
- strength
- weight
- future health

Eating On The Go

It's easier than you think to make good choices at a fast-food restaurant, the mall, or even the school cafeteria. Most cafeterias and fast-food places offer healthy choices that are also tasty, like grilled chicken or salads. Be mindful of portion sizes and high fat add-ons, like dressings, sauces or cheese.

About This Chapter: Information in this chapter is excerpted from "Eating Well While Eating Out," © 1995–2016. The Nemours Foundation/KidsHealth®. Reprinted with permission.

Here are some pointers to remember that can help you make wise choices when eating out:

- **Go for balance.** Choose meals that contain a balance of lean proteins (like fish, chicken, or beans if you're a vegetarian), fruits and vegetables (fries and potato chips don't qualify as veggies!), and whole grains (like whole-wheat bread and brown rice). That's why a turkey sandwich on whole wheat with lettuce and tomato is a better choice than a cheeseburger on a white bun.

- **Watch portion sizes.** The portion sizes of American foods have increased over the past few decades so that we are now eating way more than we need. The average size of a hamburger in the 1950s was just 1.5 ounces, compared with today's hamburgers, which weigh in at 8 ounces or more.

- **Drink water or low-fat milk.** Regular sodas, juices, and energy drinks usually contain "empty" calories that you don't need—not to mention other stuff, like caffeine.

Tips For Eating At A Restaurant

Most restaurant portions are way larger than the average serving of food at home. Ask for half portions, share an entrée with a friend, or take half of your dish home.

Here are some other restaurant survival tips:

- Ask for sauces and salad dressings on the side and use them sparingly.

- Use salsa and mustard instead of mayonnaise or oil.

- Ask for olive or canola oil instead of butter, margarine, or shortening.

- Use nonfat or low-fat milk instead of whole milk or cream.

- Order baked, broiled, or grilled (not fried) lean meats including turkey, chicken, seafood, or sirloin steak.

- Salads and vegetables make healthier side dishes than french fries. Use a small amount of sour cream instead of butter if you order a baked potato.

- Choose fresh fruit instead of sugary, high-fat desserts.

Tips For Eating At The Mall Or Fast-Food Place

With a little planning, it's easy to eat healthy foods at the mall. Here are some choices:

- a single slice of veggie pizza

- grilled, not fried, sandwiches (for example, a grilled chicken breast sandwich)
- deli sandwiches on whole-grain bread
- a small hamburger
- a bean burrito
- a baked potato
- a side salad
- frozen yogurt

Choose the smaller sizes, especially when it comes to drinks and snacks. If you have a craving for something unhealthy, try sharing the food you crave with a friend. Here's another tip for eating while shopping: Don't put off eating until you're so hungry you could inhale everything in sight. Set a time to eat, then stop what you're doing to take a break, sit down, and savor the food you are eating.

Tips For Eating In The School Cafe

The suggestions for eating in a restaurant and at the mall apply to cafeteria food as well. Add vegetables and fruit whenever possible, and opt for leaner, lighter items. Choose sandwiches on whole-grain bread or a plain hamburger over fried foods or pizza. Go easy on the high-fat, low-nutrition items, such as mayonnaise and heavy salad dressings.

You might want to consider packing your own lunch occasionally. Here are some lunch items that pack a healthy punch:

- sandwiches with lean meats or fish, like turkey, chicken, tuna (made with low-fat mayo), lean ham, or lean roast beef. For variety, try other sources of protein, like peanut butter, hummus, or meatless chili. If you don't like your bread dry, choose mustard or a small amount of lite mayo.
- low-fat or nonfat milk, yogurt, or cheese
- any fruit that's in season
- raw baby carrots, green and red pepper strips, tomatoes, or cucumbers
- whole-grain breads, pita, bagels, or crackers

It can be easy to eat well, even on the run. And the good news is you don't have to eat perfectly all the time. It's OK to splurge every once in a while, as long as your food choices are generally good.

Chapter 35

Fast-Food Alternatives

Fast Food Could Actually Cost You More In The Long Run

When money is tight, it's easy to get drawn in by the words "99–cent menu." But saving bucks at the fast–food drive–through can backfire on you.

How?

Fast foods that are high in fat, calories and sugar can have long–term consequences on health.

Studies show that one–third of fast–food purchases can contain more than 1,000 calories. That's nearly half of what an average adult should consume in an entire day, depending on age and level of physical activity.

Researchers believe the high calorie count of these purchases is due to a combination of the type of food preparation (i.e., fried), high–calorie/high–fat menu choices, and larger portion sizes.

Fast Food Alternatives

Non-Starchy Vegetables and Fruits

1. Salad with low-fat dressings

About This Chapter: Information in this chapter is excerpted from "Pinching Pennies," National Heart, Lung, and Blood Institute (NHLBI), February 13, 2013; and information from "Fast-Food Alternatives," U.S. Department of Veterans Affairs (VA), March 30 2014.

2. Grilled, steamed or stir-fried veggies

3. Fresh fruits

4. Edamame, cucumber salad

Limit These Less Healthy Choices

1. Cream veggies, cheese vegetables

2. Mayonnaise-based salads

3. Fried or tempura veggies

4. Fruits canned in sugar or syrup

5. Salads with fried or crisp noodles

Eat These Healthy Choices

Whole Grains and/or Starchy Vegetables

1. Baked potato

2. Steamed brown rice

3. Herb-seasoned squash, peas, corn, yams

4. Beans without added fat: green, kidney, black, garbanzo

5. Small whole grain bread (pumpernickel, rye)

6. Small whole grain dinner roll, English muffin, breadstick or French baguette

7. Whole grain crackers

8. Pasta primavera

Limit These Less Healthy Choices

1. French fries or onion rings

2. Fried rice

3. Butter, fried, creamed veggies

4. Refried beans and/or beans with added fat

5. Croissants

6. Biscuits, cornbread, muffins or garlic bread

7. Tortilla chips or buttered popcorn

8. Alfredo or cream sauce pasta

Eat These Healthy Choices

Lean Meat/Protein

1. Grilled, roasted, smoked chicken (white meat/no skin)

2. Grilled, boiled, broiled, baked, smoked fish

3. Fish and chicken tacos

4. Grilled, broiled sirloin, filet steak

5. Turkey, roast beef, lean ham, veggie burger, turkey burger, turkey dogs

6. Pork tenderloin, grilled lean pork

7. Steamed or baked tofu

Limit These Less Healthy Choices

1. Fried, breaded, popcorn chicken and wings

2. Fried or breaded fish

3. Beef tacos

4. Rib eye, prime rib

5. Large or double hamburgers or cheeseburgers, bologna, hot dogs, pastrami, corned beef fried pork

6. Deep-fried tofu

Combination And Miscellaneous Foods

Not everything fits neatly in the sections of the Healthy Plate, for example a lean roast beef sandwich can fit in the category of lean protein (roast beef) with the whole grain bread fitting in the healthy grain section. Here are some combo foods and some miscellaneous items that do not fit perfectly in a section of the Healthy Plate.

Table 35.1. Combination And Miscellaneous Foods

Eat These Healthy Choices	Limit These Less Healthy Choices
Stir fry with vegetables and lean meat	Pot pies
Pasta primavera or vegetable pasta salad	Macaroni and cheese
Thin-crust veggie pizza with less cheese	Meat-lovers pizza, thick-crust or butter-crust pizza with extra cheese
Meatless, low-fat cheese lasagna	Meat and cheese lasagna
Stuffed bell peppers with lean beef	Shepherd's pie
Egg on English muffin	Burrito with steak
Whole grain 6-inch sub–more veggies, less sauces	Foot-long sub with cheese and sauces
Antipasto with vegetables	Antipasto with meat
Dairy:	
Free (skim) or low-fat (1%) varieties of:	
Milk fat	Whole milk (4% fat)
Cottage cheese	Cottage cheese (4% fat)
Cheese	Cheeses
Sherbet, sorbet	Ice cream
Yogurt parfait	Milkshake
Appetizers:	
Clear or tomato-based soups	Chowder or cream soups
Salad with low-fat dressing	Mozzarella sticks
Shrimp with cocktail sauce	Nachos, onion rings, potato skins
Raw vegetable sticks	Fried/tempura vegetables
Steamed vegetable or chicken dumplings	Fried chicken wings
Egg drop, miso, wonton, or hot and sour soups	Fried egg roll or wonton
Desserts:	
Soft-serve ice cream	Sundaes
Soft-serve frozen yogurt	Cheesecake
Fruit	Banana splits
Low-fat yogurt	Fried ice cream
Sugar-free gelatin	Cakes, pies, and brownies
Sugar-free pudding	Cookies

Table 35.1. Continued

Eat These Healthy Choices	Limit These Less Healthy Choices
Beverages:	
Water, seltzer	Beer
Low-fat milk	Sugar-sweetened soda
Coffee	Sport drinks
Unsweetened tea	Sweetened tea
Sugar-free drinks	Alcoholic beverages
100% juice	Juice drinks
Condiments:	
Light dressing	Mayonnaise
Butter spray, olive oil	Butter
Pickles	Bacon bits or Chinese noodles
Mustard	Tartar sauce or mayo
Ketchup	Thousand Island dressing
Vinegar	High-calorie dips
Hot sauce	Gravy
Low-fat sour cream or fresh salsa	Sour cream
Fresh fruit jelly	Regular jelly or spreads
Sauces such as rice-wine vinegar, ponzu, wasabi, ginger, and low sodium soy sauce	Coconut milk, sweet and sour sauce, regular soy sauce

Tips For Making Healthier Fast-Food Choices

- Make careful menu selections–pay attention to menu descriptions

- Avoid dishes labeled deep-fried, pan-fried, basted, batter-dipped, breaded, creamy, crispy, scalloped, Alfredo, au gratin, or in cream sauce.

- Order items with more vegetables and choose lean proteins that are baked, broiled, or grilled rather than fried.

- Drink water with your meal

- Many beverages are a huge source of hidden calories. Try adding a little lemon to your water or ordering unsweetened iced tea.

- "Undress" your food

- Leave off the cheese and hold the mayo!

- Avoid creamy dressings, spreads, cheeses, and sour cream.

- If you add condiments, like ketchup, use small amounts.

- Do NOT Super-Size!

- Say "No" to "Would you like fries (or pie or cookies) with that?"

Chapter 36
Eating In The School Cafeteria

More than at other meals, kids have a lot of control over what they eat for lunch at school. A kid can choose to eat the green beans or throw them out. A kid also can choose to eat an apple instead of an ice cream sandwich.

When choosing what to eat for lunch, making a healthy choice is really important. Here's why: Eating a variety of healthy foods gives you energy to do stuff, helps you grow the way you should, and can even keep you from getting sick.

Think of your school lunch as the fuel you put in your tank. If you choose the wrong kind of fuel, you might run out of energy before the day is over.

To Buy Or Not To Buy

Most kids have the choice of packing lunch or buying one at school. The good news is that a kid can get a healthy lunch by doing either one. But it's not a slam-dunk. Chances are, some meals and foods served in the school cafeteria are healthier than others.

That doesn't mean you shouldn't buy your lunch, it just means you might want to give the cafeteria menu a closer look. Read the cafeteria menu the night before. Knowing what's for lunch beforehand will let you know if you want to eat it! Bring home a copy of the menu or figure out how to find it on the school website.

A packed lunch isn't automatically healthier than one you buy at school. If you pack chocolate cake and potato chips, that's not a nutritious meal! But a packed lunch, if you do it right, does have a clear advantage. When you pack your lunch, you can be sure it includes **your**

About This Chapter: Information in this chapter is excerpted from "School Lunches," © 1995–2016. The Nemours Foundation/KidsHealth®. Reprinted with permission.

favorite healthy foods—stuff you know you like. It's not a one-size-fits-all lunch. It's a lunch just for you. If your favorite sandwich is peanut butter and banana, just make it and pack it—then you can eat it for lunch. Or maybe you love olives. Go ahead and pack them!

If you want to pack your lunch, you'll need some help from your parents. Talk to them about what you like to eat in your lunch so they can stock up on those foods. Parents might offer to pack your lunch for you. This is nice of them, but you may want to watch how they do it and ask if you can start making your lunches yourself. It's a way to show that you're growing up.

10 Steps To A Great Lunch

Whether you pack or buy your lunch, follow these guidelines:

1. **Choose fruits and vegetables.** Fruits and vegetables are like hitting the jackpot when it comes to nutrition. They make your plate more colorful and they're packed with vitamins and fiber. It's a good idea to eat at least five servings of fruits and vegetables every day, so try to fit in one or two at lunch. A serving isn't a lot. A serving of carrots is ½ cup or about 6 baby carrots. A fruit serving could be one medium orange.

2. **Know the facts about fat.** Kids need some fat in their diets to stay healthy—it also helps keep you feeling full—but you don't want to eat too much of it. Fat is found in butter, oils, cheese, nuts, and meats. Some higher-fat lunch foods include french fries, hot dogs, cheeseburgers, macaroni and cheese, and chicken nuggets. Don't worry if you like these foods! No food is bad, but you may want to eat them less often and in smaller portions. Foods that are lower in fat are usually baked or grilled. Some of the best low-fat foods are fruits, vegetables, and skim and low-fat milk.

3. **Let whole grains reign.** "Grains" include breads, cereals, rice, and pasta. But as we learn more about good nutrition, it's clear that whole grains are better than refined grains. What's the difference? Brown rice is a whole grain, but white rice is not. Likewise, whole-wheat bread contains whole grains, whereas regular white bread does not.

4. **Slurp sensibly.** It's not just about what you eat—drinks count, too! Milk has been a favorite lunchtime drink for a long time. If you don't like milk, choose water. Avoid juice drinks and sodas.

5. **Balance your lunch.** When people talk about balanced meals, they mean meals that include a mix of food groups: some grains, some fruits, some vegetables, some meat or protein foods, and some dairy foods such as milk and cheese. Try to do this with your

lunch. If you don't have a variety of foods on your plate, it's probably not balanced. A double order of french fries, for example, would not make for a balanced lunch.

6. **Steer clear of packaged snacks.** Many schools make salty snacks, candy, and soda available in the cafeteria or in vending machines. It's OK to have these foods once in a while, but they shouldn't be on your lunch menu.

7. **Mix it up.** Do you eat the same lunch every day? If that lunch is a hot dog, it's time to change your routine. Keep your taste buds from getting bored and try something new. Eating lots of different kinds of food gives your body a variety of nutrients.

8. **Quit the clean plate club.** Because lunch can be a busy time, you might not stop to think whether you're getting full. Try to listen to what your body is telling you. If you feel full, it's OK to stop eating.

9. **Use your manners.** Cafeterias sometimes look like feeding time at the zoo. Don't be an animal! Follow those simple rules your parents are always reminding you about: Chew with your mouth closed. Don't talk and eat at the same time. Use your utensils. Put your napkin on your lap. Be polite. And don't make fun of what someone else is eating.

10. **Don't drink milk and laugh at the same time!** Whatever you do at lunch, don't tell your friends a funny joke when they're drinking milk. Before you know it, they'll be laughing and that milk will be coming out their noses! Gross!

Chapter 37
Healthy Snacking

Some Smart Snacks For Teens

Many adults think that snacking isn't a healthy habit for their growing teen. The truth is that most teens need snacks; the trick is making healthy food choices in the right amounts. Eating too many calories can cause teens to become overweight, which puts them at higher risk for getting type 2 diabetes Teens can lower their risk for the disease if they stay at a healthy weight by being active and choosing the right amounts of healthy foods–including snacks.

Type 2 diabetes used to be called "adult diabetes" but now more teens are getting type 2 diabetes, especially if they are overweight. Healthy snacking can be part of an overall eating plan. When your teen is making snacks, encourage him or her to use a small plate or bowl and to snack at the table instead of in front of the TV or computer. These habits help teens control portion size and take their time while eating so they don't eat too much. Be active as a family by going on walks together and encourage your teen to join active youth recreation programs.

Help your teen choose healthy snacks using these smart ideas:

1. Make a fruit pizza. Spread 2 tablespoons of nonfat cream cheese on a toasted English muffin. Top with 1/4 cup of sliced strawberries, handful of grapes, or 1/4 cup of any fruit canned in its own juice. Instead of fruit, you can also use broccoli, carrots, and tomatoes for a veggie twist.

2. Choose one small bag or handful of baked chips pretzels, or air-popped popcorn.

About This Chapter: Information in this chapter is excerpted from "Ten Smart Snacks for Teens," National Institute of Diabetes and Digestive and Kidney Diseases (NIDDK), June 2013; and information from "Choosing Foods for Your Family," We Can!®, National Heart, Lung, and Blood Institute (NHLBI), May 17, 2013.

3. Make a homemade fruit smoothie. Mix a 1/2 cup of frozen vanilla yogurt, a 1/2 cup of 100 percent orange juice, and one peeled orange in a blender then serve.

4. Serve two rice cakes, six whole-grain crackers, or one slice of whole-grain bread with 2 tablespoons of low-fat cheese, fruit spread, hummus, or peanut butter.

5. Choose an individual serving size of sugar-free, nonfat pudding instead of regular ice cream.

6. Serve a small tortilla with one or two slices of low-fat cheese or turkey, or a small bowl of vegetable soup and a few crackers.

7. Pour nonfat or low-fat milk over 1 cup of whole-grain cereal and add 1/4 cup of blueberries, strawberries, or peaches.

8. Spread 1 tablespoon of peanut butter on a tortilla and then sprinkle 1 tablespoon of whole-grain cereal on top. Peel and place one banana on the tortilla and then roll the tortilla for a crunchy treat.

9. Try an apple, banana, or plum with one or two reduced-fat or low-fat string cheese sticks.

10. Mix 1/8 cup of almonds and 1/8 cup of dried cranberries, cherries, or raisins with 1/2 cup of whole-grain cereal for a fun trail mix.

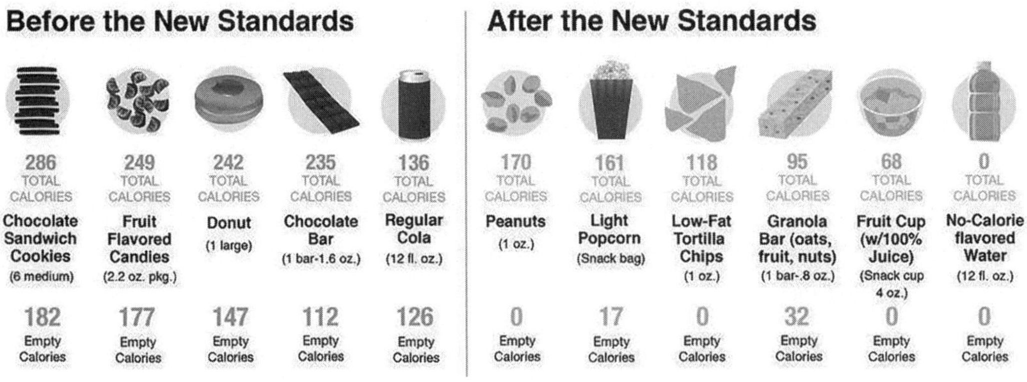

Figure 37.1. Healthy Snacking

Source: "Focusing on Smart Snacks," U.S. Department of Agriculture (USDA), August 17, 2016

GO, SLOW, and WHOA Foods

An easy way to learn about which foods are lower in fat and calories is to think in terms of GO, SLOW, and WHOA.

GO Foods Are:

- Lowest in fat and sugar
- Relatively low in calories
- "Nutrient dense" (rich in vitamins, minerals, and other nutrients important to health)
- Great to eat anytime

Examples include:

- Fruits and vegetables
- Whole grains
- Fat-free or low-fat milk and milk products
- Lean meat, poultry, fish
- Beans, eggs, and nuts

SLOW Foods Are:

- Higher in fat, added sugar, and calories
- To be eaten sometimes/less often

WHOA Foods Are:

- Highest in fat and added sugar
- "Calorie-dense" (high in calories)
- Often low in nutrients
- To be eaten only once in a while/on special occasions, in small portions

Chapter 38

What You Should Know About Caffeine And Energy Drinks

What Is Caffeine?

Caffeine is a drug that is naturally produced in the leaves and seeds of many plants. It's also produced artificially and added to certain foods. Caffeine is defined as a drug because it stimulates the central nervous system, causing increased alertness. Caffeine gives most people a temporary energy boost and elevates mood.

Caffeine is in tea, coffee, chocolate, many soft drinks, and pain relievers and other over-the-counter medications. In its natural form, caffeine tastes very bitter. But most caffeinated drinks have gone through enough processing to camouflage the bitter taste.

Teens usually get most of their caffeine from soft drinks and energy drinks. (In addition to caffeine, these also can have added sugar and artificial flavors.) Caffeine is not stored in the body, but you may feel its effects for up to 6 hours.

Got The Jitters?

Many people feel that caffeine increases their mental alertness. Higher doses of caffeine can cause anxiety, dizziness, headaches, and the jitters. Caffeine can also interfere with normal sleep.

Caffeine sensitivity (the amount of caffeine that will produce an effect in someone) varies from person to person. On average, the smaller the person, the less caffeine needed to produce side effects. Caffeine sensitivity is most affected by the amount of caffeine a person has daily.

About This Chapter: Information in this chapter is excerpted from "Caffeine," © 1995–2016. The Nemours Foundation/ KidsHealth ®. Reprinted with permission; information from "The Buzz on Energy Drinks," Healthy Schools, Centers for Disease Control and Prevention (CDC), March 22, 2016; and information from "Alcohol and Public Health," Centers for Disease Control and Prevention (CDC), November 12, 2015.

People who regularly take in a lot of caffeine soon develop less sensitivity to it. This means they may need more caffeine to achieve the same effects.

Caffeine is a mild diuretic, meaning it causes a person to urinate (pee) more. Drinking a moderate amount of caffeine isn't likely to cause dehydration, but it's probably a good idea to stay away from too much caffeine in hot weather, during long workouts, or in other situations where you might sweat a lot.

Caffeine also may cause the body to lose calcium, and that can lead to bone loss over time. Drinking caffeine-containing soft drinks and coffee instead of milk can have an even greater impact on bone density and the risk of developing osteoporosis.

Caffeine can aggravate certain heart problems. It also may interact with some medicines or supplements. If you are stressed or anxious, caffeine can make these feelings worse. Although caffeine is sometimes used to treat migraine headaches, it can make headaches worse for some people.

Moderation Is The Key

Caffeine is usually thought to be safe in moderate amounts. Experts consider 200–300 mg of caffeine a day to be a moderate amount for adults. But consuming as little as 100 mg of caffeine a day can lead a person to become "dependent" on caffeine. This means that someone may develop withdrawal symptoms (like tiredness, irritability, and headaches) if he or she quits caffeine suddenly.

Teens should try to limit caffeine consumption to no more than 100 mg of caffeine daily, and kids should get even less. The following chart includes common caffeinated products and the amounts of caffeine they contain:

Table 38.1. Common Caffeinated Products And The Amounts Of Caffeine

Drink/Food/ Supplement	Amount of Drink/Food	Amount of Caffeine
SoBe No Fear	8 ounces	83 mg
Monster energy drink	16 ounces	160 mg
Rockstar energy drink	8 ounces	80 mg
Red Bull energy drink	8.3 ounces	80 mg
Jolt cola	12 ounces	72 mg
Mountain Dew	12 ounces	55 mg
Coca-Cola	12 ounces	34 mg
Diet Coke	12 ounces	45 mg

Table 38.1. Continued

Drink/Food/ Supplement	Amount of Drink/Food	Amount of Caffeine
Pepsi	12 ounces	38 mg
7-Up	12 ounces	0 mg
Brewed coffee (drip method)	5 ounces	115 mg*
Iced tea	12 ounces	70 mg*
Cocoa beverage	5 ounces	4 mg*
Chocolate milk beverage	8 ounces	5 mg*
Dark chocolate	1 ounce	20 mg*
Milk chocolate	1 ounce	6 mg*
Jolt gum	1 stick	33 mg
Cold relief medication	1 tablet	30 mg*
Vivarin	1 tablet	200 mg
Excedrin extra strength	2 tablets	130 mg

*denotes average amount of caffeine

Cutting Back

If you're taking in too much caffeine, you may want to cut back. The best way is to cut back slowly. Otherwise, you could get headaches and feel tired, irritable, or just plain lousy.

Try cutting your intake by replacing caffeinated sodas and coffee with noncaffeinated drinks, like water, decaffeinated coffee, caffeine-free sodas, and caffeine-free teas. Start by keeping track of how many caffeinated drinks you have each day, then substitute one of these daily drinks with a caffeine-free alternative. Continue this for a week. Then, if you are still drinking too much caffeine, substitute another of your daily drinks, again, keeping it up for a week. Do this for as many weeks as it takes to bring your daily caffeine intake below the 100-milligram mark. Taking a gradual approach like this can help you wean yourself from caffeine without unwanted side effects like headaches.

As you cut back on the amount of caffeine you consume, you may find yourself feeling tired. Be sure you're getting enough sleep and boost your energy by exercising. As your body adjusts to less caffeine, your energy levels should return to normal in a few days.

What Is An Energy Drink?

- A beverage that typically contains large amounts of caffeine, added sugars, other additives, and legal stimulants such as guarana, taurine, and L-carnitine. These legal stimulants can increase alertness, attention, energy, as well as increase blood pressure, heart rate, and breathing.

- These drinks are often used by students to provide an extra boost in energy. However, the stimulants in these drinks can have a harmful effect on the nervous system.

Energy Drink Recommendations For Adolescents

- The American Academy of Pediatrics recommends that adolescents do not consume energy drinks, yet between 30% and 50% reported consuming energy drinks.
- The National Federation of State High School Associations recommends that young athletes should not use energy drinks for hydration, and information about the potential risk should be widely distributed to young athletes.

The Potential Dangers Of Energy Drinks

Some of the dangers of energy drinks include

- dehydration (not enough water in your body)

- heart complications (such as irregular heartbeat and heart failure)

- anxiety (feeling nervous and jittery)

- insomnia (unable to sleep)

Dangers Of Mixing Alcohol With Energy Drinks

- Energy drinks are beverages that typically contain caffeine, other plant-based stimulants, simple sugars, and other additives. They are very popular among young people and are regularly consumed by 31 percent of 12- to 17-year-olds and 34 percent of 18- to 24-year-olds.

- When alcoholic beverages are mixed with energy drinks, a popular practice among young people, the caffeine in these drinks can mask the depressant effects of alcohol. At the same time, caffeine has no effect on the metabolism of alcohol by the liver and thus does not reduce breath alcohol concentrations or reduce the risk of alcohol-attributable harms.

- Drinkers who consume alcohol mixed with energy drinks are 3 times more likely to binge drink (based on breath alcohol levels) than drinkers who do not report mixing alcohol with energy drinks.

- Drinkers who consume alcohol with energy drinks are about twice as likely as drinkers who do not report mixing alcohol with energy drinks to report being taken advantage of sexually, to report taking advantage of someone else sexually, and to report riding with a driver who was under the influence of alcohol.

Fast Facts: Are Kids Getting These Drinks At School?

- While nationally only 1.2 percent of high schools sell energy drinks a la carte to students in the cafeteria, as many as 11.6 percent of secondary schools in some districts sell energy drinks in vending machines, school stores, and snack bars.
- Nationwide, 75 percent of school districts do not have a policy in place regarding these types of beverages that contain high levels of caffeine for sale in vending machines, schools stores, or a la carte in the cafeteria.

Chapter 39

Sports Supplements

If you're a competitive athlete or a fitness buff, improving your sports performance is probably on your mind. Lots of people wonder if taking sports supplements could offer fast, effective results without so much hard work. But do sports supplements really work? And are they safe?

What Are Sports Supplements?

Sports supplements (also called **ergogenic aids**) are products used to enhance athletic performance that may include vitamins, minerals, amino acids, herbs, or botanicals (plants)—or any concentration, extract, or combination of these. These products are generally available over the counter without a prescription.

Sports supplements are considered dietary supplements. Dietary supplements do not require U.S. Food and Drug Administration (FDA) approval before they come on the market. Supplement manufacturers do have to follow the FDA's current good manufacturing practices to ensure quality and safety of their product, though. And the FDA is responsible for taking action if a product is found to be unsafe after it has gone on the market.

Critics of the supplement industry point out cases where manufacturers haven't done a good job of following standards. They also mention instances where the FDA hasn't enforced regulations. Both of these can mean that supplements contain variable amounts of ingredients or even ingredients not listed on the label.

Some over-the-counter medicines and prescription medications, including anabolic steroids, are used to enhance performance but they are not considered supplements. Although

About This Chapter: Information in this chapter is excerpted from "Sports Supplements," © 1995–2016. The Nemours Foundation/KidsHealth®. Reprinted with permission.

medications are FDA approved, using medicines—even over-the-counter ones—in ways other than their intended purpose puts the user at risk of serious side effects. For example, teen athletes who use medications like human growth hormone (hGH) that haven't been prescribed for them can have problems with growth, and may develop diabetes and heart problems.

Lots of sports organizations have developed policies on sports supplements. The National Football League (NFL), the National Collegiate Athletic Association (NCAA), and the International Olympic Committee (IOC) have banned the use of steroids, ephedra, and androstenedione by their athletes, and competitors who use them face fines, ineligibility, and suspension from their sports.

The National Federation of State High School Associations (NFHS) strongly recommends that student athletes consult with their doctor before taking any supplement.

How Some Common Supplements Affect The Body?

Whether you hear about sports supplements from your teammates in the locker room or the sales clerk at your local vitamin store, chances are you're not getting the whole story about how supplements work, if they are really effective, and the risks you take by using them.

Androstenedione And DHEA

Androstenedione (also known as andro) and dehydroepiandrosterone (also known as DHEA) are prohormones or "natural steroids" that can be broken down into testosterone. Andro used to be available over the counter, but now requires a prescription.

When researchers studied these prohormones in adult athletes, DHEA and andro did not increase muscle size, improve strength or enhance performance.

Andro and DHEA can cause hormone imbalances in people who use them. Both can have the same effects as taking anabolic steroids and may lead to dangerous side effects like testicular cancer, infertility, stroke, and an increased risk of heart disease. As with anabolic steroids, teens who use andro while they are still growing may not reach their full adult height. Natural steroid supplements can also cause breast development and shrinking of testicles in guys.

Creatine

Creatine is already manufactured by the body in the liver, kidneys, and pancreas. It also occurs naturally in foods such as meat and fish. Creatine supplements are available over the counter.

People who take creatine usually take it to improve strength, but the long-term and short-term effects of creatine use haven't been studied in teens and kids. Research in adults found that creatine is most effective for athletes doing intermittent high-intensity exercise with short recovery intervals, such as sprinting and power lifting. However, researchers found no effect on athletic performance in nearly a third of athletes studied. Creatine has not been found to increase endurance or improve aerobic performance.

The most common side effects of creatine supplements include weight gain, diarrhea, abdominal pain, and muscle cramps. People with kidney problems should not use creatine because it may affect kidney function. The American College of Sports Medicine recommends that people younger than 18 years old do not use creatine. If you are considering using creatine, talk with your doctor about the risks and benefits, as well as appropriate dosing.

Fat Burners

Fat burners (sometimes known as **thermogenics**) were often made with an herb called ephedra, also known as ephedrine or ma huang, which acts as a stimulant and increases metabolism. Some athletes use fat burners to lose weight or to increase energy—but ephedra-based products can be one of the most dangerous supplements. Evidence has shown that it can cause heart problems, stroke, and occasionally even death.

Because athletes and others have died using this supplement, ephedra has been taken off the market. Since the ban, "ephedra-free" products have emerged, but they often contain ingredients with ephedra-like properties, including bitter orange or country mallow. Similar to ephedra, these supplements can cause high blood pressure, heart attack, stroke, and seizures.

Many of these products also contain caffeine, along with other caffeine sources (such as yerba mate and guarana). This combination may lead to restlessness, anxiety, racing heart, irregular heart beat, and increases the chance of having a life-threatening side effect.

Will Supplements Make Me A Better Athlete?

Sports supplements haven't been tested on teens and kids. But studies on adults show that the claims of many supplements are weak at best. Most won't make you any stronger, and none will make you any faster or more skillful.

Many factors go into your abilities as an athlete—including your diet, how much sleep you get, genetics and heredity, and your training program. But the fact is that using sports supplements may put you at risk for serious health conditions.

So instead of turning to supplements to improve your performance, concentrate on nutrition and training, including strength and conditioning programs.

Tips For Dealing With Athletic Pressure And Competition

Ads for sports supplements often use persuasive before and after pictures that make it look easy to get a muscular, toned body. But the goal of supplement advertisers is to make money by selling more supplements, and many claims may be misleading.

Teens and kids may seem like an easy sell on supplements because they may feel dissatisfied or uncomfortable with their still-developing bodies, and many supplement companies try to convince teens that supplements are an easy solution.

Don't waste your money on expensive and dangerous supplements. Instead, try these tips for getting better game:

- **Make downtime a priority.** Studies show that teens need more than 8 hours of sleep a night, and sleep is important for athletes. Organize time for sleep into your schedule by doing as much homework as possible on the weekend or consider cutting back on after-school job hours during your sports season.

- **Learn to relax.** Your school, work, and sports schedules may have you sprinting from one activity to the next, but taking a few minutes to relax can be helpful. Meditating or visualizing your success during the next game may improve your performance; sitting quietly and focusing on your breathing can give you a brief break and prepare you for your next activity.

- **Choose good eats.** Fried, fatty, or sugary foods will interfere with your performance. Instead, focus on eating foods such as lean meats, whole grains, vegetables, fruits, and low-fat dairy products. Celebrating with the team at the local pizza place after a big game is fine once in a while. But for most meals and snacks, choose healthy foods to keep your weight in a healthy range and your performance at its best.

- **Get enough fuel.** Sometimes people skip breakfast or have an early lunch, then try to play a late afternoon game. Not getting enough food to fuel an activity can quickly wear you out—and even place you at risk for injury or muscle fatigue. Be sure to eat lunch on practice and game days. If you feel hungry before the game, pack easy-to-carry, healthy snacks in your bag, such as fruit, trail mix, or string cheese. It's important to eat well after a workout.

- **Avoid harmful substances.** Smoking will diminish your lung capacity and your ability to breathe, alcohol can make you sluggish and tired, and can impair your hand-eye coordination and reduce your alertness. And you can kiss your team good-bye if you get caught using drugs or alcohol—many schools have a no-tolerance policy for harmful substances.

- **Train harder and smarter.** If you get out of breath easily during your basketball game and you want to increase your endurance, work on improving your cardiovascular conditioning. If you think more leg strength will help you excel on the soccer field, consider weight training to increase your muscle strength. Before changing your program, though, get advice from your doctor.

- **Consult a professional.** If you're concerned about your weight or whether your diet is helping your performance, talk to your doctor or a registered dietitian who can evaluate your nutrition and steer you in the right direction. Coaches can help too. And if you're still convinced that supplements will help you, talk to your doctor or a sports medicine specialist. The doc will be able to offer alternatives to supplements based on your body and sport.

Chapter 40

Healthy Eating For Vegans And Vegetarians

You probably know some vegetarians, or perhaps you're one yourself. But the term "vegetarian" can mean different things to different people:

- A true vegetarian eats no meat at all, including poultry and fish.

- A lacto-ovo vegetarian eats dairy products and eggs, but excludes meat, fish, and poultry.

- A lacto vegetarian eats dairy products but not eggs.

- An ovo vegetarian eats eggs but not dairy products.

And lots of people won't eat red meat or pork but do eat poultry and/or seafood.

Less commonly practiced is the form of vegetarianism known as veganism. A vegan doesn't consume **any** animal-derived foods or use animal products or byproducts, and eats only plant-based foods.

In addition to not eating meat, poultry, seafood, eggs, or dairy, vegans avoid using products made from animal sources, such as fur, leather, and wool.

While those are obvious animal products, many animal byproducts are things we might not even realize come from animals. These include:

- gelatin (made using meat byproducts)

- lanolin (made from wool)

About This Chapter: Information in this chapter is excerpted from "Vegan Food Guide," © 1995–2016. The Nemours Foundation/KidsHealth®. Reprinted with permission; and information from "Healthy Eating for Vegetarians," ChooseMyPlate.gov, U.S. Department of Agriculture (USDA), July 11, 2016.

- rennet (an enzyme found in the stomach of calves, young goats, and lambs that's used in cheese-making)

- honey and beeswax (made by bees)

- silk (made by silkworms)

- shellac (the resinous secretion of the tiny lac insect)

- cochineal (a red dye derived from the cochineal insect)

Why Vegan?

Veganism (also known as strict vegetarianism or pure vegetarianism), as defined by the Vegan Society, is "a philosophy and way of living which seeks to exclude—as far as is possible and practical—all forms of exploitation of, and cruelty to, animals for food, clothing, or any other purpose."

Vegans also avoid toothpaste with calcium extracted from animal bones, if they are aware of it. Similarly, soap made from animal fat rather than vegetable fats is avoided. Vegans generally oppose the violence and cruelty involved in the meat, dairy, cosmetics, clothing, and other industries.

What About Nutrition?

According to the Academy of Nutrition and Dietetics (AND), "appropriately planned vegetarian diets, including total vegetarian or vegan diets, are healthful, nutritionally adequate and may provide health benefits in the prevention and treatment of certain diseases. Well-planned vegetarian diets are appropriate for individuals during all stages of the life-cycle including pregnancy, lactation, infancy, childhood and adolescence and for athletes."

Vegetarian diets offer a number of advantages, including lower levels of total fat, saturated fat, and cholesterol, and higher levels of fiber, magnesium, potassium, folate, and antioxidants. As a result, the health benefits of a vegetarian diet may include the prevention of certain diseases, including heart disease, diabetes, and some cancers.

But any restrictive diet can make it more difficult to get all the nutrients your body needs. A vegan diet eliminates food sources of vitamin B12, which is found almost exclusively in animal products, including milk, eggs, and cheese. A vegan diet also eliminates milk products, which are good sources of calcium.

Getting What You Need

To ensure that "well-planned" diet, vegans must find alternative sources for B12 and calcium, as well as vitamin D, protein, iron, zinc, and occasionally riboflavin.

Here's how:

Vitamin B12. Vegans can get vitamin B12, needed to produce red blood cells and maintain normal nerve function, from enriched breakfast cereals, fortified soy products, nutritional yeast, or supplements.

Calcium. We all need calcium for strong teeth and bones. You can get calcium from dark green vegetables (spinach, bok choy, broccoli, collards, kale, turnip greens), sesame seeds, almonds, red and white beans, soy foods, dried figs, blackstrap molasses, and calcium-fortified foods like soy, rice, and almond milks; fruit juices; and breakfast cereals.

Vitamin D. Vitamin D helps our bodies absorb calcium and is synthesized by exposing skin to sunlight. But vitamin D deficiency can occur, especially if you don't spend a lot of time outside. Vitamin D is not found in most commonly eaten plant foods; the best dietary sources are fortified dairy products. Vegans also can get vitamin D from fortified foods, including vitamin D-fortified soy milk, rice milk, almond milk, orange juice, and some cereals. Vitamin D2 supplements are plant-derived, whereas most vitamin D3 is derived from animal products.

Protein. Not getting enough protein is a concern when switching to a vegetarian diet. Protein needs can be met while following a vegan diet if you consume adequate calories and eat a variety of plant foods, including good plant sources of protein such as soy, other legumes, nuts, and seeds.

Iron. Iron from plant sources is less easily absorbed than iron in meat. This lower bioavailability means that iron intake for vegetarians should be higher than the RDA for nonvegetarians. Vegetarian food sources of iron include soy foods like soybeans, tempeh, and tofu; legumes like lentils and chickpeas; and fortified cereals. Iron absorption is enhanced by vitamin C.

Zinc. Zinc plays a role in many key body functions, including immune system response, so it's important to get enough of it, which vegans can do by eating nuts, legumes, miso and other soy products, pumpkin and sunflower seeds, tahini, wheat germ, and whole-grain breads and cereals.

Omega-3 fatty acids. The omega 3 fatty acids (DHA, EPA, and ALA) are important for cardiovascular health and brain function. DHA and EPA are found in fish, eggs, and algae. Vegans can get these essential fatty acids through a diet rich in alpha linolenic acid (ALA), a plant-based omega-3 fatty acid. ALA is found in flaxseed, chia seed, walnuts, canola oil, soy. DHA from microalgae can be found in supplements and fortified foods.

Eating A Vegan Diet

Anyone following a vegan diet has to be a meticulous label-reader. No federal regulation dictates the use of the words "vegetarian" or "vegan" in the United States. To be sure a food truly is "suitable for vegans," check the label—what might be vegetarian isn't necessarily vegan.

Vegans are by no means stuck eating boring foods with little variety. But if you're considering becoming a vegan, or wondering whether it's realistic to eliminate animal-based foods from your diet, it might pay to start slowly, especially if you've been a cheeseburger fan most of your life.

Try some of the wide array of meat alternatives that are found in almost every grocery store. Tasty frozen veggie burgers, chicken and meat substitutes, sausage alternative, fake bacon, and tofu dogs will make the transition to a vegan diet convenient and easy.

If you need help, talk to a registered dietician familiar with vegan diets and look for vegetarian cookbooks that can help you plan and prepare healthy meatless meals.

And remember, many foods you probably already have are suitable for a vegan diet. For instance, most breakfast cereals are vegan as are many crackers, cookies, and baked goods. Choose ones made with whole grains and low in fat, pair them with healthy salads, fresh fruits, and some colorful veggies, and you might not ever miss that ham and cheese sandwich!

Healthy Eating For Vegetarians

A vegetarian eating pattern can be a healthy option. The key is to consume a variety of foods and the right amount of foods to meet your calorie and nutrient needs.

- **Think about protein.** Your protein needs can easily be met by eating a variety of plant foods. Sources of protein for vegetarians include beans and peas, nuts, and soy products (such as tofu, tempeh). Lacto-ovo vegetarians also get protein from eggs and dairy foods.

- **Bone up on sources of calcium.** Calcium is used for building bones and teeth. Some vegetarians consume dairy products, which are excellent sources of calcium. Other sources of calcium for vegetarians include calcium-fortified soymilk (soy beverage), tofu made with calcium sulfate, calcium-fortified breakfast cereals and orange juice, and some dark-green leafy vegetables (collard, turnip, and mustard greens; and bok choy).

- **Make simple changes.** Many popular main dishes are or can be vegetarian—such as pasta primavera, pasta with marinara or pesto sauce, veggie pizza, vegetable lasagna, tofu-vegetable stir-fry, and bean burritos.

- **Enjoy a cookout.** For barbecues, try veggie or soy burgers, soy hot dogs, marinated tofu or tempeh, and fruit kabobs. Grilled veggies are great, too!

- **Include beans and peas.** Because of their high nutrient content, consuming beans and peas is recommended for everyone, vegetarians and non-vegetarians alike. Enjoy some vegetarian chili, three bean salad, or split pea soup. Make a hummus filled pita sandwich.

- **Try different veggie versions.** A variety of vegetarian products look—and may taste—like their non-vegetarian counterparts but are usually lower in saturated fat and contain no cholesterol. For breakfast, try soy-based sausage patties or links. For dinner, rather than hamburgers, try bean burgers or falafel (chickpea patties).

- **Make some small changes at restaurants.** Most restaurants can make vegetarian modifications to menu items by substituting meatless sauces or nonmeat items, such as tofu and beans for meat, and adding vegetables or pasta in place of meat. Ask about available vegetarian options.

- **Nuts make great snacks.** Choose unsalted nuts as a snack and use them in salads or main dishes. Add almonds, walnuts, or pecans instead of cheese or meat to a green salad.

- **Get your vitamin B12.** Vitamin B12 is naturally found only in animal products. Vegetarians should choose fortified foods such as cereals or soy products, or take a vitamin B12 supplement if they do not consume any animal products. Check the Nutrition Facts label for vitamin B12 in fortified products.

Part Five
Eating And Weight-Related Concerns

Chapter 41
Body Mass Index For Teens

What Is Body Mass Index (BMI)?

Body mass index (BMI) is a person's weight in kilograms divided by the square of height in meters. For teens, BMI is age- and sex-specific and is often referred to as BMI-for-age.

A high BMI can be an indicator of high body fatness. BMI does not measure body fat directly, but research has shown that BMI is correlated with more direct measures of body fat, such as skinfold thickness measurements, bioelectrical impedance, densitometry (underwater weighing), dual energy X-ray absorptiometry (DXA) and other methods. BMI can be considered an alternative to direct measures of body fat. In general, BMI is an inexpensive and easy-to-perform method of screening for weight categories that may lead to health problems.

How Is BMI Calculated for Teens?

Calculating BMI using the BMI Percentile Calculator (nccd.cdc.gov/dnpabmi/Calculator. aspx) involves the following steps:

1. Measure height and weight.

2. Use the Child and Teen BMI Calculator (nccd.cdc.gov/dnpabmi/Calculator.aspx) to calculate BMI. The BMI number is calculated using standard formulas.

About This Chapter: Information in this chapter is excerpted from "About Child and Teen BMI," Centers for Disease Control and Prevention (CDC), May 15, 2015.

What Is A BMI Percentile And How Is It Interpreted?

After BMI is calculated for children and teens, it is expressed as a percentile which can be obtained from either a graph or a percentile calculator. These percentiles express a child's BMI relative to children in the United States who participated in national surveys that were conducted from 1963–65 to 1988–94. Because weight and height change during growth and development, as does their relation to body fatness, a child's BMI must be interpreted relative to other children of the same sex and age.

The BMI-for-age percentile growth charts are the most commonly used indicator to measure the size and growth patterns of teens in the United States. BMI-for-age weight status categories and the corresponding percentiles were based on expert committee recommendations and are shown in the following table.

Table 41.1. Percentile Range

Weight Status Category	Percentile Range
Underweight	Less than the 5th percentile
Normal or Healthy Weight	5th percentile to less than the 85th percentile
Overweight	85th to less than the 95th percentile
Obese	Equal to or greater than the 95th percentile

How Is BMI Used With Teens?

For teens, BMI is not a diagnostic tool and is used to screen for potential weight and health-related issues.

Is BMI Interpreted The Same Way For Teens As It Is For Adults?

BMI is interpreted differently for teens even though it is calculated as weight ÷ height. Because there are changes in weight and height with age, as well as their relation to body fatness, BMI levels among teens need to be expressed relative to other children of the same sex and age. These percentiles are calculated from the Centers for Disease Control and Prevention (CDC) growth charts, which were based on national survey data collected from 1963–65 to 1988–94.

Obesity is defined as a BMI at or above the 95th percentile for teens of the same age and sex.

Why Can't Healthy Weight Ranges Be Provided For Teens?

Normal or healthy weight weight status is based on BMI between the 5th and 85th percentile on the CDC growth chart. It is difficult to provide healthy weight ranges for teens because the interpretation of BMI depends on weight, height, age, and sex.

What Are The BMI Trends For Teens In The United States?

The prevalence of teens who measure in the 95th percentile or greater on the CDC growth charts has greatly increased over the past 40 years. Recently, however, this trend has leveled off and has even declined in certain age groups.

How Can I Tell If My Child Is Overweight Or Obese?

CDC and the American Academy of Pediatrics (AAP) recommend the use of BMI to screen for overweight and obesity in children and teens age 2 through 19 years. Although BMI is used to screen for overweight and obesity in teens, BMI is not a diagnostic tool. To determine whether the child has excess fat, further assessment by a trained health professional would be needed.

Can I Determine If My Teen Is Obese By Using An Adult BMI Calculator?

In general, it's not possible to do this.

The adult calculator provides only the BMI value (weight/height^2) and not the BMI percentile that is needed to interpret BMI among children and teens. It is not appropriate to use the BMI categories for adults to interpret the BMI of children and teens.

However, if a child or teen has a BMI of ≥ 30 kg/m^2, the child is almost certainly obese. A BMI of 30 kg/m^2 is approximately the 95th percentile among 17-year-old girls and 18-year-old boys.

My Two Children Have The Same BMI Values, But One Is Considered Obese And The Other Is Not. Why Is That?

The interpretation of BMI varies by age and sex. So if the children are not the same age and the same sex, the interpretation of BMI has different meanings. For children of different age and sex, the same BMI could represent different BMI percentiles and possibly different weight status categories.

See the following graphic for an example for a 10-year-old boy and a 15-year-old boy who both have a BMI-for-age of 23. (Note that two children of different ages are plotted on the same growth chart to illustrate a point. Normally the measurement for only one child is plotted on a growth chart.)

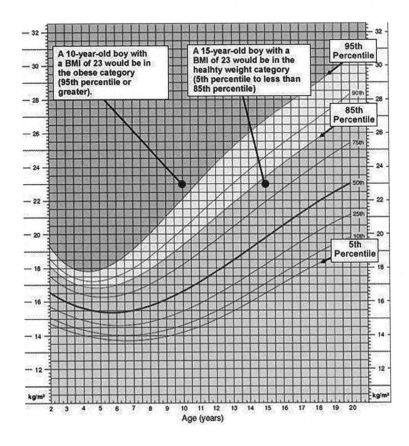

Figure 41.1. Body Mass Index-For-Age Percentiles: Boys, 2 to 20 Years

Chapter 42
What's The Right Weight For My Height?

"What's the right weight for my height?" is one of the most common questions girls and guys have. It seems like a simple question. But, for teens, it's not always an easy one to answer.

It's normal for two people who are the same height and age to have very different weights. First, not everyone goes through puberty at the same time: Some kids start developing as early as age 8 and others might not develop until age 14. Second, people have different body types. Some are more muscular or shaped differently than others.

You can't point to a number on a scale as the "right" number, but it is possible to find out if you are in a *healthy weight range* for your height and age. That's why doctors use BMI.

People Grow And Develop Differently

Not everyone grows and develops on the same schedule, but most people go through a period of faster growth during their teens. During puberty, the body begins making hormones that spark physical changes like faster muscle growth (particularly in guys) and spurts in height. As the amount of muscle, fat, and bone in the body changes during this time, some people might gain weight more rapidly.

It can feel strange adjusting to a new body. But all that new weight gain can be perfectly fine—as long as body fat, muscle, and bone are in the right proportion.

About This Chapter: Information in this chapter is excerpted from "What's the Right Weight for My Height?" © 1995–2016. The Nemours Foundation/KidsHealth®. Reprinted with permission.

Figuring Out Fat Using BMI

Because weight is more complicated during our teens, doctors don't rely on weight alone to figure out if someone is in a healthy weight range. Instead, they use the body mass index, or BMI. **BMI is a formula that doctors use to estimate how much body fat a person has based on his or her weight and height.**

The BMI formula uses height and weight measurements to calculate a BMI number. This number is then plotted on a BMI chart, which helps tell a person whether he or she is in the underweight, healthy weight, overweight, or obese range.

The growth charts have lines for "percentiles." Like percentages, percentiles go from 0 to 100. The eight lines on the BMI growth charts show the 5th, 10th, 25th, 50th, 75th, 85th, 90th, and 95th percentiles. The 50th percentile line is the average BMI of the teens who were measured to make the chart.

When your BMI is plotted on the chart, the doctor can see how you compare with other people the same age and gender as you. Based on where your number is on the chart, a doctor will decide if your BMI is in the underweight, normal weight, overweight, or obese range.

There's a big range of normal on the chart: Anyone who falls between the 5th percentile and the 85th percentile is in the healthy weight range. If someone is at or above the 85th percentile line on the chart (but less than the 95th percentile), that person may be overweight. A BMI measurement over the 95th percentile line on the chart puts someone in the obese range.

What Does BMI Tell Us?

You can calculate BMI on your own, but it's a good idea to ask your doctor, school nurse, or other health professional to help you figure out what it means.

A doctor can use BMI results from past years to track whether you may be at risk for becoming overweight. Spotting this risk early on can be helpful because the person can then make changes in diet and exercise to help head off a weight problem.

BMI can be a good indicator of a person's body fat, but it doesn't always tell the full story. People can have a high BMI because they have a large frame or a lot of muscle (like a bodybuilder or athlete) instead of excess fat. Likewise, a small person with a small frame might have a normal BMI but could still have too much body fat. These are other good reasons to talk about your BMI with your doctor.

How Can I Be Sure I'm Not Overweight Or Underweight?

If you think you've gained too much weight or you're too skinny, a doctor can help you decide whether it's normal for you or whether you really have a weight problem. **Your doctor has measured your height and weight and has plotted your BMI over time. So he or she can tell whether you're growing normally.**

If your doctor is concerned about your height, weight, or BMI, he or she may ask questions about your health, physical activity, and eating habits. Your doctor also may ask about your family background to find out if you've inherited traits that might make you taller, shorter, or a late bloomer (someone who develops later than other people the same age). The doctor can then put all this information together to decide whether you might have a weight or growth problem.

If your doctor thinks you're overweight, he or she may refer you to a dietitian or doctor specializing in weight management. These experts can offer eating and exercise recommendations based on your individual needs. Following a doctor's or dietitian's plan that's designed especially for you will work way better than following fad diets.

What if you're worried about being too skinny? **Most teens who weigh less than other people their age are just fine.** You might be going through puberty on a different schedule than some of your peers, and your body may be growing and changing at a different rate. Most underweight teens catch up eventually and there's rarely a need to try to gain weight.

In a few cases, teens can be underweight because of a health problem that needs treatment. See a doctor if you notice any of these things:

- You feel tired or ill a lot.

- You have a cough, stomachache, diarrhea, or other problems that have lasted for more than a week orv two.

Some people are underweight because of eating disorders, like anorexia or bulimia, that they need to get help for.

Getting Into Your Genes

Heredity plays a role in body shape and what a person weighs. People from different races, ethnic groups, and nationalities tend to have different body fat distribution (meaning they have fat in different parts of their bodies) or body composition (their amounts of bone and muscle versus fat).

But genes are not destiny. No matter whose genes you inherit, you can have a healthy body and keep your weight at a level that's normal for you by eating right and being active.

Genes aren't the only things that family members may share. Unhealthy eating habits can be passed down, too. The eating and exercise habits of people in the same household may have an even greater effect than genes on a person's risk of becoming overweight.

If your family eats a lot of high-fat foods or snacks or doesn't get much exercise, you may tend to do the same. The good news is these habits can be changed for the better. Even simple changes like walking more or taking the stairs can benefit a person's health.

It can be tough dealing with the physical changes your body goes through during puberty. But at this time, more than any other, it's not a specific number on the scale that's important. It's keeping your body healthy—inside and out.

Chapter 43
Body Image And Self-Esteem

Does any of this sound familiar? "I'm too tall." "I'm too short." "I'm too skinny." "If only I were shorter/taller/had curly hair/straight hair/a smaller nose/longer legs, I'd be happy."

Are you putting yourself down? If so, you're not alone. As a teen, you're going through lots of changes in your body. And, as your body changes, so does your image of yourself. It's not always easy to like every part of your looks, but when you get stuck on the negatives it can really bring down your self-esteem.

Why Are Self-Esteem And Body Image Important?

Self-esteem is all about how much you feel you are worth—and how much you feel other people value you. Self-esteem is important because feeling good about yourself can affect your mental health and how you behave.

People with high self-esteem know themselves well. They're realistic and find friends that like and appreciate them for who they are. People with high self-esteem usually feel more in control of their lives and know their own strengths and weaknesses.

Body image is how you view your physical self—including whether you feel you are attractive and whether others like your looks. For many people, especially people in their early teens, body image can be closely linked to self-esteem.

What Influences A Person's Self-Esteem?

Puberty And Development

Some people struggle with their self-esteem and body image when they begin puberty because it's a time when the body goes through many changes. These changes, combined with wanting to feel accepted by our friends, means it can be tempting to compare ourselves with others. The trouble with that is, not everyone grows or develops at the same time or in the same way.

Media Images And Other Outside Influences

Our tweens and early teens are a time when we become more aware of celebrities and media images—as well as how other kids look and how we fit in. We might start to compare ourselves with other people or media images ("ideals" that are frequently airbrushed). All of this can affect how we feel about ourselves and our bodies even as we grow into our teens.

Families And School

Family life can sometimes influence our body image. Some parents or coaches might be too focused on looking a certain way or "making weight" for a sports team. Family members might struggle with their own body image or criticize their kids' looks ("why do you wear your hair so long?" or "how come you can't wear pants that fit you?"). This can all influence a person's self-esteem, especially if they're sensitive to others peoples' comments.

People also may experience negative comments and hurtful teasing about the way they look from classmates and peers. Although these often come from ignorance, sometimes they can affect body image and self-esteem.

Healthy Self-Esteem

If you have a positive body image, you probably like and accept yourself the way you are, even if you don't fit some media "ideal." This healthy attitude allows you to explore other aspects of growing up, such as developing good friendships, becoming more independent from your parents, and challenging yourself physically and mentally. Developing these parts of yourself can help boost your self-esteem.

A positive, optimistic attitude can help people develop strong self-esteem. For example, if you make a mistake, you might want to say, "Hey, I'm human" instead of "Wow, I'm such a loser" or not blame others when things don't go as expected.

Knowing what makes you happy and how to meet your goals can help you feel capable, strong, and in control of your life. A positive attitude and a healthy lifestyle (such as exercising and eating right) are a great combination for building good self-esteem.

Tips For Improving Body Image

Some people think they need to change how they look to feel good about themselves. But all you need to do is change the way you see your body and how you think about yourself. Here are some tips on doing that:

Recognize that your body is your own, no matter what shape or size it comes in. Try to focus on how strong and healthy your body is and the things it can do, not what's wrong with it or what you feel you want to change about it. If you're worried about your weight or size, check with your doctor to verify that things are OK. But it's no one's business but your own what your body is like—ultimately, you have to be happy with yourself.

Identify which aspects of your appearance you can realistically change and which you can't. Humans, by definition, are imperfect. It's what makes each of us unique and original! Everyone (even the most perfect-seeming celeb) has things that they can't change and need to accept—like their height, for example, or their shoe size. Remind yourself that "real people aren't perfect and perfect people aren't real (they're usually airbrushed!)".

If there are things about yourself that you want to change and can, do this by making goals for yourself. For example, if you want to get fit, make a plan to exercise every day and eat healthy. Then keep track of your progress until you reach your goal. Meeting a challenge you set for yourself is a great way to boost self-esteem!

When you hear negative comments coming from within, tell yourself to stop. Appreciate that each person is more than just how he or she looks on any given day. We're complex and constantly changing. Try to focus on what's unique and interesting about yourself.

Try building your self-esteem by giving yourself three compliments every day. While you're at it, every evening list three things in your day that really gave you pleasure. It can be anything from the way the sun felt on your face, the sound of your favorite band, or the way someone laughed at your jokes. By focusing on the good things you do and the positive aspects of your life, you can change how you feel about yourself.

Some people with physical disabilities or differences may feel they are not seen for their true selves because of their bodies and what they can and can't do. Other people may have such serious body image issues that they need a bit more help. Working with a counselor or therapist can help some people gain perspective and learn to focus on their individual strengths as well as develop healthier thinking.

Where Can I Go If I Need Help?

Sometimes low self-esteem and body image problems are too much to handle alone. A few teens may become depressed, and lose interest in activities or friends. Some go on to develop eating disorders or body image disorders, or use alcohol or drugs to escape feelings of low worth.

If you're feeling this way, it can help to talk to a parent, coach, religious leader, guidance counselor, therapist, or friend. A trusted adult—someone who supports you and doesn't bring you down—can help you put your body image in perspective and give you positive feedback about your body, your skills, and your abilities.

If you can't turn to anyone you know, call a teen crisis hotline (an online search can give you the information for national and local hotlines). The most important thing is to get help if you feel like your body image and self-esteem are affecting your life.

Chapter 44

Weight-Loss And Nutrition Myths

"Lose 30 pounds in 30 days!"

"Eat as much as you want and still lose weight!"

"Try the thigh buster and lose inches fast!"

Have you heard these claims before? A large number of diets and tools are available, but their quality may vary. It can be hard to know what to believe.

This chapter may help. Here, we discuss myths and provide facts and tips about weight loss, nutrition, and physical activity. This information may help you make healthy changes in your daily habits. You can also talk to your healthcare provider. She or he can help you if you have other questions or you want to lose weight. A registered dietitian may also give you advice on a healthy eating plan and safe ways to lose weight and keep it off.

Weight-loss And Diet Myths

Myth: Fad diets will help me lose weight and keep it off.

Fact: Fad diets are not the best way to lose weight and keep it off. These diets often promise quick weight loss if you strictly reduce what you eat or avoid some types of foods. Some of these diets may help you lose weight at first. But these diets are hard to follow. Most people quickly get tired of them and regain any lost weight.

Fad diets may be unhealthy. They may not provide all of the nutrients your body needs. Also, losing more than 3 pounds a week after the first few weeks may increase your chances of

About This Chapter: Information in this chapter is excerpted from "Weight-Loss and Nutrition Myths," National Institute of Diabetes and Digestive and Kidney Diseases (NIDDK), October 2014.

developing gallstones (solid matter in the gallbladder that can cause pain). Being on a diet of fewer than 800 calories a day for a long time may lead to serious heart problems.

TIP: Research suggests that safe weight loss involves combining a reduced-calorie diet with physical activity to lose 1/2 to 2 pounds a week (after the first few weeks of weight loss). Make healthy food choices. Eat small portions. Build exercise into your daily life. Combined, these habits may be a healthy way to lose weight and keep it off. These habits may also lower your chances of developing heart disease, high blood pressure, and type 2 diabetes.

Myth: Grain products such as bread, pasta, and rice are fattening. I should avoid them when trying to lose weight.

Fact: A grain product is any food made from wheat, rice, oats, cornmeal, barley, or another cereal grain. Grains are divided into two subgroups, whole grains and refined grains. Whole grains contain the entire grain kernel—the bran, germ, and endosperm. Examples include brown rice and whole-wheat bread, cereal, and pasta. Refined grains have been milled, a process that removes the bran and germ. This is done to give grains a finer texture and improve their shelf life, but it also removes dietary fiber, iron, and many B vitamins.

People who eat whole grains as part of a healthy diet may lower their chances of developing some chronic diseases. Government dietary guidelines advise making half your grains whole grains. For example, choose 100 percent whole-wheat bread instead of white bread, and brown rice instead of white rice.

TIP: To lose weight, reduce the number of calories you take in and increase the amount of physical activity you do each day. Create and follow a healthy eating plan that replaces less healthy options with a mix of fruits, veggies, whole grains, protein foods, and low-fat dairy:

- Eat a mix of fat-free or low-fat milk and milk products, fruits, veggies, and whole grains.
- Limit added sugars, cholesterol, salt (sodium), and saturated fat.
- Eat low-fat protein: beans, eggs, fish, lean meats, nuts, and poultry.

Meal Myths

Myth: Some people can eat whatever they want and still lose weight.

Fact: To lose weight, you need to burn more calories than you eat and drink. Some people may seem to get away with eating any kind of food they want and still lose weight. But those people, like everyone, must use more energy than they take in through food and drink to lose weight.

A number of factors such as your age, genes, medicines, and lifestyle habits may affect your weight. If you would like to lose weight, speak with your healthcare provider about factors that may affect your weight. Together, you may be able to create a plan to help you reach your weight and health goals.

Eat The Rainbow!

When making half of your plate fruits and veggies, choose foods with vibrant colors that are packed with fiber, minerals, and vitamins.

Red: bell peppers, cherries, cranberries, onions, red beets, strawberries, tomatoes, watermelon

Green: avocado, broccoli, cabbage, cucumber, dark lettuce, grapes, honeydew, kale, kiwi, spinach, zucchini

Orange and yellow: apricots, bananas, carrots, mangoes, oranges, peaches, squash, sweet potatoes

Blue and purple: blackberries, blueberries, grapes, plums, purple cabbage, purple carrots, purple potatoes

TIP: When trying to lose weight, you can still eat your favorite foods as part of a healthy eating plan. But you must watch the **total number of calories** that you eat. Reduce your portion sizes. Find ways to limit the calories in your favorite foods. For example, you can bake foods rather than frying them. Use low-fat milk in place of cream. Make half of your plate fruits and veggies.

Myth: "Low-fat" or "fat-free" means no calories.

Fact: A serving of low-fat or fat-free food may be lower in calories than a serving of the full-fat product. But many processed low-fat or fat-free foods have just as many calories as the full-fat versions of the same foods—or even more calories. These foods may contain added flour, salt, starch, or sugar to improve flavor and texture after fat is removed. These items add calories.

TIP: Read the Nutrition Facts label on a food package to find out how many calories are in a serving. Check the serving size, too—it may be less than you are used to eating.

Myth: Fast foods are always an unhealthy choice. You should not eat them when dieting.

Fact: Many fast foods are unhealthy and may affect weight gain. However, if you do eat fast food, choose menu options with care. Both at home and away, choose healthy foods that are nutrient rich, low in calories, and small in portion size.

TIP: To choose healthy, low-calorie options, check the nutrition facts. These are often offered on the menu or on restaurant websites. And know that the nutrition facts often do not include sauces and extras. Try these tips:

- Avoid "value" combo meals, which tend to have more calories than you need in one meal.

- Choose fresh fruit items or nonfat yogurt for dessert.

- Limit your use of toppings that are high in fat and calories, such as bacon, cheese, regular mayonnaise, salad dressings, and tartar sauce.

- Pick steamed or baked items over fried ones.

- Sip on water or fat-free milk instead of soda.

Myth: If I skip meals, I can lose weight.

Fact: Skipping meals may make you feel hungrier and lead you to eat more than you normally would at your next meal. In particular, studies show a link between skipping breakfast and obesity. People who skip breakfast tend to be heavier than people who eat a healthy breakfast.

TIP: Choose meals and snacks that include a variety of healthy foods. Try these examples:

- For a quick breakfast, make oatmeal with low-fat milk, topped with fresh berries. Or eat a slice of whole-wheat toast with fruit spread.

- Pack a healthy lunch each night, so you won't be tempted to rush out of the house in the morning without one.

- For healthy nibbles, pack a small low-fat yogurt, a couple of whole-wheat crackers with peanut butter, or veggies with hummus.

Myth: Eating healthy food costs too much.

Fact: Eating better does not have to cost a lot of money. Many people think that fresh foods are healthier than canned or frozen ones. For example, some people think that spinach is better for you raw than frozen or canned. However, canned or frozen fruits and veggies provide as many nutrients as fresh ones, at a lower cost. Healthy options include low-salt canned veggies and fruit canned in its own juice or water-packed. Remember to rinse canned veggies to remove excess salt. Also, some canned seafood, like tuna, is easy to keep on the shelf, healthy, and low-cost. And canned, dried, or frozen beans, lentils, and peas are also healthy sources of protein that are easy on the wallet.

TIP: Check the nutrition facts on canned, dried, and frozen items. Look for items that are high in calcium, fiber, potassium, protein, and vitamin D. Also check for items that are low in added sugars, saturated fat, and sodium.

Food Myths

Myth: Eating meat is bad for my health and makes it harder to lose weight.

Fact: Eating lean meat in small amounts can be part of a healthy plan to lose weight. Chicken, fish, pork, and red meat contain some cholesterol and saturated fat. But they also contain healthy nutrients like iron, protein, and zinc.

TIP: Choose cuts of meat that are lower in fat, and trim off all the fat you can see. Meats that are lower in fat include chicken breast, pork loin and beef round steak, flank steak, and extra lean ground beef. Also, watch portion size. Try to eat meat or poultry in portions of 3 ounces or less. Three ounces is about the size of a deck of cards.

Myth: Dairy products are fattening and unhealthy.

Fact: Fat-free and low-fat cheese, milk, and yogurt are just as healthy as whole-milk dairy products, and they are lower in fat and calories. Dairy products offer protein to build muscles and help organs work well, and calcium to strengthen bones. Most milk and some yogurts have extra vitamin D added to help your body use calcium. Most Americans don't get enough calcium and vitamin D. Dairy is an easy way to get more of these nutrients.

TIP: Based on Government guidelines, you should try to have 3 cups a day of fat-free or low-fat milk or milk products. This can include soy beverages fortified with vitamins. If you can't digest lactose (the sugar found in dairy products), choose lactose-free or low-lactose dairy products or other foods and beverages that have calcium and vitamin D:

- calcium: soy-based beverages or tofu made with calcium sulfate; canned salmon; dark leafy greens like collards or kale
- vitamin D: cereals or soy-based beverages

Myth: "Going vegetarian" will help me lose weight and be healthier.

Fact: Research shows that people who follow a vegetarian eating plan, on average, eat fewer calories and less fat than non-vegetarians. Some research has found that vegetarian-style eating patterns are associated with lower levels of obesity, lower blood pressure, and a reduced risk of heart disease.

Vegetarians also tend to have lower body mass index (BMI) scores than people with other eating plans. (The BMI measures body fat based on a person's height in relation to weight). But

245

vegetarians—like others—can make food choices that impact weight gain, like eating large amounts of foods that are high in fat or calories or low in nutrients.

The types of vegetarian diets eaten in the United States can vary widely. Vegans do not consume any animal products, while lacto-ovo vegetarians eat milk and eggs along with plant foods. Some people have eating patterns that are mainly vegetarian but may include small amounts of meat, poultry, or seafood.

TIP: If you choose to follow a vegetarian eating plan, be sure you get enough of the nutrients that others usually take in from animal products such as cheese, eggs, meat, and milk. Nutrients that may be lacking in a vegetarian diet are listed in the sidebar, along with foods and beverages that may help you meet your body's needs for these nutrients.

Table 44.1. Nutrient And Common Sources

Nutrient	Common Sources
Calcium	Dairy products, soy beverages with added calcium, tofu made with calcium sulfate, collard greens, kale, broccoli
Iron	Cashews, spinach, lentils, chickpeas, bread or cereal with added iron
Protein	Eggs, dairy products, beans, peas, nuts, seeds, tofu, tempeh, soy-based burgers
Vitamin B12	Eggs, dairy products, fortified cereal or soy beverages, tempeh, miso (tempeh and miso are foods made from soybeans)
Vitamin D	Foods and beverages with added vitamin D, including milk, soy beverages, or cereal
Zinc	Whole grains (check the ingredients list on product labels for the words "whole" or "whole grain" before the grain ingredient's name), nuts, tofu, leafy greens (spinach, cabbage, lettuce)

Chapter 45

Choosing A Safe And Successful Weight-Loss Program

Do you need to lose weight? Have you been thinking about trying a weight-loss program? Diets and programs that promise to help you lose weight are advertised everywhere—through magazines and newspapers, radio, TV, and websites. Are these programs safe? Will they work for you?

This chapter provides tips on how to identify a weight-loss program that may help you lose weight safely and keep the weight off over time. It also suggests ways to talk to your healthcare provider about your weight. He or she may be able to help you control your weight by making changes to your eating and physical activity habits. If these changes are not enough, you may want to consider a weight-loss program or other types of treatment.

Where Do I Start?

Talking to your healthcare provider about your weight is an important first step. Doctors do not always address issues such as healthy eating, physical activity, and weight control during general office visits. It is important for you to bring up these issues to get the help you need. Even if you feel uneasy talking about your weight with your doctor, remember that he or she is there to help you improve your health.

Prepare for the visit:

• Write down your questions in advance.

• Bring pen and paper to take notes.

• Invite a family member or friend along for support if this will make you feel better.

About This Chapter: Information in this chapter is excerpted from "Choosing a Safe and Successful Weight-Loss Program," National Institute of Diabetes and Digestive and Kidney Diseases (NIDDK), December 2012. Reviewed September 2016.

Talk to your doctor about safe and effective ways to control your weight.

He or she can review any medical problems that you have and any drugs that you take to help you set goals for controlling your weight. Make sure you understand what your doctor is saying. Ask questions if you do not understand something.

You may want to ask your doctor to recommend a weight-loss program or specialist. If you do start a weight-loss program, discuss your choice of program with your doctor, especially if you have any health problems.

What Should I Look For In A Weight-Loss Program?

Successful, long-term weight control must focus on your overall health, not just on what you eat. Changing your lifestyle is not easy, but adopting healthy habits may help you manage your weight in the long run.

Effective weight-loss programs include ways to keep the weight off for good. These programs promote healthy behaviors that help you lose weight and that you can stick with every day.

Safe and effective weight-loss programs should include

- a plan to keep the weight off over the long run

- guidance on how to develop healthier eating and physical activity habits

- ongoing feedback, monitoring, and support

- slow and steady weight-loss goals—usually 1/2 to 2 pounds per week (though weight loss may be faster at the start of a program)

Some weight-loss programs may use very low-calorie diets (up to 800 calories per day) to promote rapid weight loss among people who have a lot of excess weight. This type of diet requires close medical supervision through frequent office visits and medical tests.

What If The Program Is Offered Online?

Many weight-loss programs are now being offered online—either fully or partly. Not much is known about how well these programs work. However, experts suggest that online weight-loss programs should provide the following:

- Structured, weekly lessons offered online or by podcasts support tailored to your personal goals

- Support tailored to your personal goals

- Self-monitoring of eating and physical activity using handheld devices, such as cell phones or online journals

- Regular feedback from a counselor on goals, progress, and results, given by email, phone, or text messages

- Social support from a group through bulletin boards, chat rooms, and/or online meetings

Whether the program is online or in person, you should get as much background as you can before deciding to join.

What Questions Should I Ask About The Program?

Professionals working for weight-loss programs should be able to answer questions about the program's features, safety, costs, and results. The following are sample questions you may want to ask.

What Does The Weight-Loss Program Include?

- Does the program offer group classes or one-on-one counseling that will help me develop healthier habits?

- Do I have to follow a specific meal plan or keep food records?

- Do I have to buy special meals or supplements?

- If the program requires special foods, can I make changes based on my likes, dislikes, and food allergies (if any)?

- Will the program help me be more physically active, follow a specific physical activity plan, or provide exercise guidelines?

- Will the program work with my lifestyle and cultural needs? Does the program provide ways to deal with such issues as social or holiday eating, changes to work schedules, lack of motivation, and injury or illness?

- Does the program include a plan to help me keep the weight off once I've lost weight?

What Are The Staff Credentials?

- Who supervises the program?

- What type of weight-control certifications, education, experience, and training do the staff have?

Does The Product Or Program Carry Any Risks?

- Could the program hurt me?

- Could the suggested drugs or supplements harm my health?

- Do the people involved in the program get to talk with a doctor?

- Does a doctor or other certified health professional run the program?

- Will the program's doctor or staff work with my healthcare provider if needed (for example, to address how the program may affect an existing medical issue)?

- Is there ongoing input and follow-up from a healthcare provider to ensure my safety while I take part in the program?

How Much Does The Program Cost?

- What is the total cost of the program?

- Are there other costs, such as membership fees, fees for weekly visits, and payments for food, meal replacements, supplements, or other products?

- Are there other fees for medical tests?

- Are there fees for a follow-up program after I lose weight?

What Results Do People In The Program Typically Have?

- How much weight does the average person lose?

- How long does the average person keep the weight off?

- Do you have written information on these results?

If it seems too good to be true...it probably is!

In choosing a weight-loss program, watch out for these false claims:

- Lose weight without diet or exercise!
- Lose weight while eating all of your favorite foods!
- Lose 30 pounds in 30 days!
- Lose weight in specific problem areas of your body!

Other warning signs include

- Very small print
- Asterisks and footnotes
- Before-and-after photos that seem too good to be true

Chapter 46
Should I Gain Weight?

Why Do People Want To Gain Weight?

Some of the reasons people give for wanting to gain weight are:

I'm worried that there's something wrong with me. If you want to gain weight because you think you have a medical problem, talk to your doctor. Although certain health conditions can cause a person to be underweight, most of them have symptoms other than skinniness, like stomach pain or diarrhea. So it's likely that if some kind of medical problem is making you skinny, you probably wouldn't feel well.

I'm worried because all of my friends have filled out and I haven't. Many guys and girls are skinny until they start to go through puberty. The changes that come with puberty include weight gain and, in guys, broader shoulders and increased muscle mass.

Because everyone is on a different schedule, some of your friends may have started to fill out when they were as young as 8 (if they're girls) or 9 (if they're guys). But for some normal kids, puberty may not start until 12 or later for girls and 14 or later for guys. And whenever you start puberty, it may take 3 or 4 years for you to fully develop and gain all of the weight and muscle mass you will have as an adult.

Some people experience what's called delayed puberty. If you are one of these "late bloomers," you may find that some relatives of yours developed late, too. Most teens who have delayed puberty don't need to do anything; they'll eventually develop normally—and that includes gaining weight and muscle. If you are concerned about delayed puberty, though, talk to your doctor.

I've always wanted to play a certain sport; now I don't know if I can. Lots of people come to love a sport in grade school or middle school—and then find themselves on the bench later when their teammates develop faster. If you've always envisioned yourself playing football, it can be tough when your body doesn't seem to want to measure up. You may need to wait until your body goes through puberty before you can play football on the varsity squad.

Another option to consider is switching your ambitions to another sport. If you were the fastest defensive player on your middle school football team but now it seems that your body type is long and lean, maybe track and field is for you. Many adults find that the sports they love the most are those that fit their body types the best.

I just hate the way I look! Developing can be tough enough without the pressure to be perfect. Your body changes (or doesn't change), your friends' bodies change (or don't), and you all spend a lot of time noticing. It's easy to judge both yourself and others based on appearances. Sometimes, it can feel like life is some kind of beauty contest!

Your body is your own, and as frustrating as it may seem to begin with, there are certain things you can't speed up or change. But there is one thing you can do to help: Work to keep your body healthy so that you can grow and develop properly. Self-esteem can play a part here, too. People who learn to love their bodies and accept them for what they are carry themselves well and project a type of self-confidence that helps them look attractive.

If you're having trouble with your body image, talk about how you feel with someone you like and trust who's been through it—maybe a parent, doctor, counselor, coach, or teacher.

It's The Growth, Not The Gain

No matter what your reason is for wanting to gain weight, here's a simple fact: The majority of teens have no reason—medical or otherwise—to try to gain weight. An effort like this will at best simply not work and at worst increase your body fat, putting you at risk for health problems.

So focus on growing strong, not gaining weight. Keeping your body healthy and fit so that it grows well is an important part of your job as a teen. Here are some things you can do to help this happen:

Make nutrition your mission. Your friends who want to slim down are eating more salads and fruit. Here's a surprise: So should you. You can do more for your body by eating a variety of healthier foods instead of trying to pack on weight by forcing yourself to eat a lot of unhealthy high-fat, high-sugar foods. Chances are, trying to force-feed yourself won't help you gain weight anyway, and if you do, you'll mostly just be gaining excess body fat.

Eating a variety of healthy foods, making time for regular meals and snacks, and eating only until you are full will give your body its best chance to stay healthy as it gets the fuel and nutrients it needs.

Good nutrition doesn't have to be complicated. Here are some simple tips:

- Eat lots of vegetables and fruits.

- Choose whole grains.

- Eat breakfast every day.

- Eat healthy snacks.

- Limit less nutritious foods, like chips and soda.

Eating well at this point in your life is important for many reasons. Good nutrition is a key part of normal growth and development. It's also wise to learn good eating habits now—they'll become second nature, which will help you stay healthy and fit without even thinking about it.

Healthy Habits Matter

Keep on moving. Another way to keep your body healthy is to incorporate exercise into your routine. This can include walking to school, playing Frisbee with your friends, or helping out with some household chores. Or you might choose to work out at a gym or with a sports team.

A good rule of thumb for exercise amounts during the teen years: Try to get at least 60 minutes of moderate to vigorous physical activity every day.

Strength training, when done safely, is a healthy way to exercise, but it won't necessarily bulk you up. Guys especially get more muscular during puberty, but puberty is no guarantee that you'll turn into a cover model for *Muscle and Fitness* in a couple of years—some people just don't have the kind of body type for this to happen. Our genes play an important role in determining our body type. Adult bodies come in all different shapes and sizes, and some people stay lean their entire lives, no matter what they do.

> If you've hit puberty, the right amount of strength training will help your muscles become stronger and have more endurance. And, once a boy has reached puberty, proper weight training can help him bulk up, if that's the goal. Girls can benefit from strength training, too, but they won't bulk up like boys.

Be sure to work with a certified trainer or other qualified adult who can show you how to do it without injuring yourself.

Get the skinny on supplements. Thinking about drinking something from a can or taking a pill to turn you buff overnight? Guess what: Supplements or pills that make promises like this are at best a waste of money and at worst potentially harmful to your health.

> The best way to get the fuel you need to build muscle is by eating well. Before you take any kind of supplement at all, even if it's just a vitamin pill, talk to your doctor.

Sleep your way to stunning. Sleep is an important component of normal growth and development. If you get enough, you'll have the energy to fuel your growth. Your body is at work while it sleeps—oxygen moves to the brain, growth hormones are released, and your bones keep on developing, even while you're resting.

Focus on feeling good. It can help to know that your body is likely to change in the months and years ahead. Few of us look like we did at 15 when we're 25. But it's also important to realize that feeling good about yourself can make you more attractive to others, too.

Chapter 47

Health Fraud Awareness

How To Spot Health Fraud

You don't have to look far to find a health product that's totally bogus—or a consumer who's totally unsuspecting. Promotions for fraudulent products show up daily in newspaper and magazine ads and TV "infomercials." They accompany products sold in stores, on the Internet, and through mail-order catalogs. They're passed along by word-of-mouth.

And consumers respond, spending billions of dollars a year on fraudulent health products, according to Stephen Barrett, M.D., head of Quackwatch Inc., a nonprofit corporation that combats health fraud. Hoping to find a cure for what ails them, improve their well-being, or just look better, consumers often fall victim to products and devices that do nothing more than cheat them out of their money, steer them away from useful, proven treatments, and possibly do more bodily harm than good.

"There's a lot of money to be made," says Bob Gatling, director of the program operations staff in the U.S. Food and Drug Administration's (FDA) Center for Devices and Radiological Health. "People want to believe there's something that can cure them."

FDA describes health fraud as "articles of unproven effectiveness that are promoted to improve health, well being or appearance." The articles can be drugs, devices, foods, or cosmetics for human or animal use.

FDA shares federal oversight of health fraud products with the Federal Trade Commission (FTC). FDA regulates safety, manufacturing and product labeling, including claims in

About This Chapter: Information in this chapter is excerpted from "How to Spot Health Fraud," U.S. Food and Drug Administration (FDA), May 5, 2016; and information from "6 Tip-offs to Rip-offs: Don't Fall for Health Fraud Scams," U.S. Food and Drug Administration (FDA), May 10, 2016.

labeling, such as package inserts and accompanying literature. FTC regulates advertising of these products.

Because of limited resources, says Joel Aronson, team leader for the nontraditional drug compliance team in FDA's Center for Drug Evaluation and Research, the agency's regulation of health fraud products is based on a priority system that depends on whether a fraudulent product poses a direct or indirect risk.

When the use of a fraudulent product results in injuries or adverse reactions, it's a direct risk. When the product itself does not cause harm but its use may keep someone away from proven, sometimes essential, medical treatment, the risk is indirect. For example, a fraudulent product touted as a cure for diabetes might lead someone to delay or discontinue insulin injections or other proven treatments.

While FDA remains vigilant against health fraud, many fraudulent products may escape regulatory scrutiny, maintaining their hold in the marketplace for some time to lure increasing numbers of consumers into their web of deceit.

How can you avoid being scammed by a worthless product? Though health fraud marketers have become more sophisticated about selling their products, Aronson says, these charlatans often use the same old phrases and gimmicks to gain consumers' attention—and trust. You can protect yourself by learning some of their techniques.

Tip-Offs To Rip-offs

FDA offers some tip-offs to help you identify rip-offs.

- One product does it all. Be suspicious of products that claim to cure a wide range of diseases. A New York firm claimed its products marketed as dietary supplements could treat or cure senile dementia, brain atrophy, atherosclerosis, kidney dysfunction, gangrene, depression, osteoarthritis, dysuria, and lung, cervical, and prostate cancer.

- Personal testimonials. Success stories, such as, "It cured my diabetes" or "My tumors are gone," are easy to make up and are not a substitute for scientific evidence.

- Quick fixes. Few diseases or conditions can be treated quickly, even with legitimate products. Beware of language such as, "Lose 30 pounds in 30 days" or "eliminates skin cancer in days."

- "All natural." Some plants found in nature (such as poisonous mushrooms) can kill when consumed. Moreover, FDA has found numerous products promoted as "all natural" but that contain hidden and dangerously high doses of prescription drug ingredients or even untested active artificial ingredients.

- "Miracle cure." Alarms should go off when you see this claim or others like it such as, "new discovery," "scientific breakthrough" or "secret ingredient." If a real cure for a serious disease were discovered, it would be widely reported through the media and prescribed by health professionals—not buried in print ads, TV infomercials or on Internet sites.

- Conspiracy theories. Claims like "The pharmaceutical industry and the government are working together to hide information about a miracle cure" are always untrue and unfounded. These statements are used to distract consumers from the obvious, common-sense questions about the so-called miracle cure.

Even with these tips, fraudulent health products are not always easy to spot. If you're tempted to buy an unproven product or one with questionable claims, check with your doctor or other health care professional first.

Joining Forces To Fight Fraud

Health fraud isn't confined to the United States only. It's worldwide, and to help combat it in North America, the United States has joined with Canada and Mexico to share knowledge and coordinate enforcement activities related to fraudulent health products, services and devices.

In announcing their decision in December 1998 to adopt the Joint Strategies Agreement, the countries agreed to:

- Share information on current trends in health fraud.

- Cooperate in detecting health fraud along borders.

- Share information about significant investigations in their country.

- Consider each others' requests to investigate domestic activities and coordinate related enforcement activities.

- Develop and distribute joint consumer and business education messages about health fraud.

Chapter 48
Physical Activity And Health

The Benefits Of Physical Activity

Regular physical activity is one of the most important things you can do for your health. It can help:

- control your weight

- reduce your risk of cardiovascular disease

- reduce your risk for type 2 diabetes and metabolic syndrome

- reduce your risk of some cancers

- strengthen your bones and muscles

- improve your mental health and mood

- improve your ability to do daily activities and prevent falls, if you're an older adult

- increase your chances of living longer

If you're not sure about becoming active or boosting your level of physical activity because you're afraid of getting hurt, the good news is that **moderate-intensity aerobic activity**, like brisk walking, is generally **safe for most people**.

Start slowly. Cardiac events, such as a heart attack, are rare during physical activity. But the risk does go up when you suddenly become much more active than usual. For example, you can put yourself at risk if you don't usually get much physical activity and then all of a sudden do

About This Chapter: Information in this chapter is excerpted from "Physical Activity and Health," Centers for Disease Control and Prevention (CDC), June 4, 2015.

vigorous-intensity aerobic activity, like shoveling snow. That's why it's important to start slowly and gradually increase your level of activity.

If you have a chronic health condition such as arthritis, diabetes, or heart disease, talk with your doctor to find out if your condition limits, in any way, your ability to be active. Then, work with your doctor to come up with a physical activity plan that matches your abilities. What's important is that you avoid being inactive. Even 60 minutes a week of moderate-intensity aerobic activity is good for you.

The bottom line is—the health benefits of physical activity far outweigh the risks of getting hurt.

If you want to know more about how physical activity improves your health, the information below gives more detail on what research studies have found.

Control Your Weight

Looking to get to or stay at a healthy weight? Both diet and physical activity play a critical role in controlling your weight. You gain weight when the calories you burn, including those burned during physical activity, are less than the calories you eat or drink. When it comes to weight management, people vary greatly in how much physical activity they need. You may need to be more active than others to achieve or maintain a healthy weight.

To maintain your weight: Work your way up to 150 minutes of moderate-intensity aerobic activity, 75 minutes of vigorous-intensity aerobic activity, or an equivalent mix of the two each week. Strong scientific evidence shows that physical activity can help you maintain your weight over time. However, the exact amount of physical activity needed to do this is not clear since it varies greatly from person to person. It's possible that you may need to do more than the equivalent of 150 minutes of moderate-intensity activity a week to maintain your weight.

To lose weight and keep it off: You will need a high amount of physical activity unless you also adjust your diet and reduce the amount of calories you're eating and drinking. Getting to and staying at a healthy weight requires both regular physical activity and a healthy eating plan. The CDC has some great tools and information about nutrition, physical activity and weight loss.

Reduce Your Risk Of Cardiovascular Disease

Heart disease and stroke are two of the leading causes of death in the United States. But following the Guidelines and getting at least 150 minutes a week (2 hours and 30 minutes) of moderate-intensity aerobic activity can put you at a lower risk for these diseases. You can reduce your risk even further with more physical activity. Regular physical activity can also lower your blood pressure and improve your cholesterol levels.

Reduce Your Risk Of Type 2 Diabetes And Metabolic Syndrome

Regular physical activity can reduce your risk of developing type 2 diabetes and metabolic syndrome. Metabolic syndrome is a condition in which you have some combination of too much fat around the waist, high blood pressure, low HDL cholesterol, high triglycerides, or high blood sugar. Research shows that lower rates of these conditions are seen with 120 to 150 minutes (2 hours to 2 hours and 30 minutes) a week of at least moderate-intensity aerobic activity. And the more physical activity you do, the lower your risk will be.

Already have type 2 diabetes? Regular physical activity can help control your blood glucose levels.

Reduce Your Risk Of Some Cancers

Being physically active lowers your risk for two types of cancer: colon and breast. Research shows that:

- Physically active people have a lower risk of colon cancer than do people who are not active.

- Physically active women have a lower risk of breast cancer than do people who are not active.

Reduce your risk of endometrial and lung cancer. Although the research is not yet final, some findings suggest that your risk of endometrial cancer and lung cancer may be lower if you get regular physical activity compared to people who are not active.

Improve your quality of life. If you are a cancer survivor, research shows that getting regular physical activity not only helps give you a better quality of life, but also improves your physical fitness.

Strengthen Your Bones And Muscles

As you age, it's important to protect your bones, joints and muscles. Not only do they support your body and help you move, but keeping bones, joints, and muscles healthy can help ensure that you're able to do your daily activities and be physically active. Research shows that doing **aerobic, muscle-strengthening, and bone-strengthening physical activity** of at least a moderately-intense level **can slow the loss of bone density** that comes with age.

Hip fracture is a serious health condition that can have life-changing negative effects, especially if you're an older adult. But research shows that people who do 120 to 300 minutes of at least moderate-intensity aerobic activity each week have a lower risk of hip fracture.

Regular physical activity helps with arthritis and other conditions affecting the joints. If you have arthritis, research shows that doing 130 to 150 (2 hours and 10 minutes to 2 hours and 30 minutes) a week of moderate-intensity, low-impact aerobic activity can not only improve your ability to manage pain and do everyday tasks, but it can also make your quality of life better.

Build strong, healthy muscles. Muscle-strengthening activities can help you increase or maintain your muscle mass and strength. Slowly increasing the amount of weight and number of repetitions you do will give you even more benefits, no matter your age.

Improve Your Mental Health And Mood

Regular physical activity can help keep your thinking, learning, and judgment skills sharp as you age. It can also reduce your risk of depression and may help you sleep better. Research has shown that doing aerobic or a mix of aerobic and muscle-strengthening activities 3 to 5 times a week for 30 to 60 minutes can give you these mental health benefits. Some scientific evidence has also shown that even lower levels of physical activity can be beneficial.

Improve Your Ability To Do Daily Activities And Prevent Falls

A functional limitation is a loss of the ability to do everyday activities such as climbing stairs, or grocery shopping.

How does this relate to physical activity? If you're a physically active middle-aged, you have a lower risk of functional limitations than people who are inactive

Already have trouble doing some of your everyday activities? Aerobic and muscle-strengthening activities can help improve your ability to do these types of tasks.

Are you an older adult who is at risk for falls? Research shows that doing **balance** and **muscle-strengthening activities** each week along with **moderate-intensity aerobic activity**, like brisk walking, can help reduce your risk of falling.

Increase Your Chances Of Living Longer

Science shows that physical activity can reduce your risk of dying early from the leading causes of death, like heart disease and some cancers. This is remarkable in two ways:

1. Only a few lifestyle choices have as large an impact on your health as physical activity. People who are physically active for about 7 hours a week have a 40 percent lower risk of dying early than those who are active for less than 30 minutes a week.

2. You don't have to do high amounts of activity or vigorous-intensity activity to reduce your risk of premature death. You can put yourself at lower risk of dying early by doing at least 150 minutes a week of moderate-intensity aerobic activity.

> **Everyone can gain the health benefits of physical activity**—age, ethnicity, shape or size do not matter.

Chapter 49
Reduce Screen Time

Limit Computer Time And Television Usage

For many of us, limiting our computer use and getting away from all screens can be a challenge. "Screen time" means television screens, computer monitors, and even the handheld devices we use for checking email, listening to music, watching TV, and playing video games on the go.

Health experts say screen time at home should be limited to two hours or less a day. The time we spend in front of the screen, unless it's work- or homework-related, could be better spent being more physically active (increasing our energy out). Kids need at least 60 minutes of physical activity on most if not all days of the week.

Research by the Henry J. Kaiser Foundation shows that setting rules about media use is hard for many parents.

In 8- to 18-year-olds:

- 28 percent said their parents set TV-watching rules

- 30 percent said their parents set rules about video game use

- 36 percent said their parents set rules about computer use

However, the same study also showed that when parents set any media rules, children's media use is **almost three hours lower** per day.

About This Chapter: Information in this chapter is excerpted from "Reduce Screen Time," National Heart, Lung, and Blood Institute (NHLBI), February 13, 2013; and information from "Technology: 5 Ways To Reboot Yourself" © 1995–2016. The Nemours Foundation/KidsHealth®. Reprinted with permission.

Other Screen-Time Statistics

Children ages 8–18 spend the following amount of time in front of the screen each day:

- approximately 7.5 hours using entertainment media
- approximately 4.5 hours watching TV
- approximately 1.5 hours on the computer
- over an hour playing video games

These data lie in stark contrast to the **25 minutes per day** that children spend reading books.

Today's youth also have the following media in their bedrooms:

More than one in three have a computer, and Internet access

- half have video game players
- more than two out of three have TVs
- those with bedroom TVs spend an hour more in front of the screen than those without TVs

(*Source*: Henry J. Kaiser Foundation, "Generation M²: Media in the Lives of 8–18 Year Olds," January 2010)

Tips To Reduce Screen Time

Technology: 5 Ways To Reboot Yourself

Raise your hand if you've sent an embarrassing text message—the message that neither you nor your friend can understand because it looks like gibberish, or the one that's accidently sent to someone who shouldn't have read it.

Did you ever think that your nighttime pings, rings, and vibrates could be the reason why?

Lack of sleep can cause you to send embarrassing texts. But more important, sending and receiving messages late at night can disrupt your sleep and leave you tired and unfocused when it's time for school. Studies show that lack of sleep, or interrupted sleep, can affect everything from your mood to your sports performance.

Sure, you want to stay connected with your friends, but how useful can you be when you're exhausted? Give your "tech" (texts, emails, calls) a rest from bedtime until your alarm clock rings so you can rest.

How can you ease out of being accessible—but sluggish—all the time to unplugging at bedtime? Here are some tips to follow at night that will help boost your energy and focus in the morning:

1. **Log off your instant messenger, Facebook, and email.** Pings in the middle of the night can interrupt your sleep—even if you don't get up to answer them. And, more than likely, if your friends see that you're logged out, they'll log out too.

2. **Turn off your cell phone (don't just set it on vibrate) when it's time for bed.** Buzzes can be just as loud as beeps or rings, especially late at night when everything else is quiet. Plus, if your friends have no one to talk to, maybe they'll be inspired to turn off their cell and catch some Zzzs, too.

3. **Get in the habit of powering off your computer—especially if it's in your room.** Sometimes just logging off your instant messenger or Facebook is not enough. Blinking lights and glowing screens can make it harder to fall and stay asleep.

4. **Get your cell phone out of your room completely.** Try charging your phone overnight in a separate room. While your cell battery is restoring, you can get the sleep you need to recharge your own battery. Having your cell in another room can reduce the chance that you'll use it during and after bedtime.

5. **Make getting enough sleep your way to look and feel good.** Getting sleep is a great way to look and feel refreshed and focused in the morning. To get the sleep you need, tell your friends you will receive your last text, email, or phone call an hour before bedtime. This way, they'll know their beeps or buzzes will have to wait.

It can be quite a challenge to go from being constantly accessible to powering down at a certain time. But sticking to a cut-off curfew for your gadgets and gizmos will help you ease into bedtime and give your brain some tech-free downtime. And if you need an excuse, just say your parents are making you do it.

Part Six
Eating And Disease

Chapter 50

Disease Prevention Through Good Eating Habits

Improving Your Eating Habits

When it comes to eating, we have strong habits. Some are good ("I always eat breakfast"), and some are not so good ("I always clean my plate"). Although many of our eating habits were established during childhood, it doesn't mean it's too late to change them.

Making sudden, radical changes to eating habits such as eating nothing but cabbage soup, can lead to short term weight loss. However, such radical changes are neither healthy nor a good idea, and won't be successful in the long run. Permanently improving your eating habits requires a thoughtful approach in which you Reflect, Replace, and Reinforce.

- **REFLECT** on all of your specific eating habits, both bad and good; and, your common triggers for unhealthy eating.

- **REPLACE** your unhealthy eating habits with healthier ones.

- **REINFORCE** your new, healthier eating habits.

About This Chapter: Information in this chapter is excerpted from "Improving Your Eating Habits," Centers for Disease Control and Prevention (CDC), May 15, 2015; information from "Calcium and Vitamin D: Important at Every Age," National Institute of Arthritis and Musculoskeletal and Skin Diseases (NIAMS), May 2015; information from "Fruit and Vegetable Consumption," National Cancer Institute (NCI), March 2015; information from "Cruciferous Vegetables and Cancer Prevention," National Cancer Institute (NCI), June 7, 2012. Reviewed September 2016; information from "Heart-healthy Eating," National Heart, Lung, and Blood Institute (NHLBI), June 22, 2016; information from "Sodium: The Facts," Centers for Disease Control and Prevention (CDC), April 2016; and information from "Toxic Substances Portal—Nitrate and Nitrite," Agency for Toxic Substances and Disease Registry, Centers for Disease Control and Prevention (CDC), November 23, 2015.

The Role Of Calcium

Calcium is needed for our heart, muscles, and nerves to function properly and for blood to clot. Inadequate calcium significantly contributes to the development of osteoporosis. Many published studies show that low calcium intake throughout life is associated with low bone mass and high fracture rates. National nutrition surveys have shown that most people are not getting the calcium they need to grow and maintain healthy bones. To find out how much calcium you need, see the Recommended Calcium Intakes (in milligrams) table below.

Table 50.1. Recommended Calcium Intakes

Life-Stage Group	mg/day
9 to 13 years old	1,300
14 to 18 years old	1,300
19 to 30 years old	1,000

Calcium Culprits

Although a balanced diet aids calcium absorption, high levels of protein and sodium (salt) in the diet are thought to increase calcium excretion through the kidneys. Excessive amounts of these substances should be avoided, especially in those with low calcium intake.

Lactose intolerance also can lead to inadequate calcium intake. Those who are lactose intolerant have insufficient amounts of the enzyme lactase, which is needed to break down the lactose found in dairy products. To include dairy products in the diet, dairy foods can be taken in small quantities or treated with lactase drops, or lactase can be taken as a pill. Some milk products on the market already have been treated with lactase.

Calcium Supplements

If you have trouble getting enough calcium in your diet, you may need to take a calcium supplement. The amount of calcium you will need from a supplement depends on how much calcium you obtain from food sources. There are several different calcium compounds from which to choose, such as calcium carbonate and calcium citrate, among others. Except in people with gastrointestinal disease, all major forms of calcium supplements are absorbed equally well when taken with food.

Calcium supplements are better absorbed when taken in small doses (500 mg or less) several times throughout the day. In many individuals, calcium supplements are better absorbed when taken with food. It is important to check supplement labels to ensure that the product meets United States Pharmacopeia (USP) standards.

A Complete Osteoporosis Program

Remember, a balanced diet rich in calcium and vitamin D is only one part of an osteoporosis prevention or treatment program. Like exercise, getting enough calcium is a strategy that helps strengthen bones at any age. But these strategies may not be enough to stop bone loss caused by lifestyle, medications, or menopause. Your doctor can determine the need for an osteoporosis medication in addition to diet and exercise.

Fruits, Vegetables, And Cancer

Fruit And Vegetable Consumption

People whose diets are rich in plant foods such as fruits and vegetables have a lower risk of getting cancers of the mouth, pharynx, larynx, esophagus, stomach, and lung, and some evidence suggests that maintaining a diet rich in plant foods also lowers the risk of cancers of the colon, pancreas, and prostate. This diet also reduces the risk of diabetes, heart disease, and hypertension, helps to reduce calorie intake, and may help to control weight.

To help prevent the aforementioned cancers and other chronic diseases, experts recommend the daily consumption of 2 to 6.5 cups of fruits and vegetables, depending on one's energy needs. This includes 1 to 2.5 cups of fruits and 1 to 4 cups of vegetables, with special emphasis on dark green and orange vegetables and legumes. There is no evidence that the popular white potato protects against cancer.

What Are Cruciferous Vegetables?

Cruciferous vegetables are part of the *Brassica* genus of plants. They include the following vegetables, among others:

- arugula
- bok choy
- broccoli
- brussels sprouts
- cabbage
- cauliflower

- collard greens

- horseradish

- kale

- radishes

- rutabaga

- turnips

- watercress

- wasabi

Why Are Cancer Researchers Studying Cruciferous Vegetables?

Cruciferous vegetables are rich in nutrients, including several carotenoids (beta-carotene, lutein, zeaxanthin); vitamins C, E, and K; folate; and minerals. They also are a good fiber source.

In addition, cruciferous vegetables contain a group of substances known as glucosinolates, which are sulfur-containing chemicals. These chemicals are responsible for the pungent aroma and bitter flavor of cruciferous vegetables.

During food preparation, chewing, and digestion, the glucosinolates in cruciferous vegetables are broken down to form biologically active compounds such as indoles, nitriles, thiocyanates, and isothiocyanates. Indole-3-carbinol (an indole) and sulforaphane (an isothiocyanate) have been most frequently examined for their anticancer effects.

Is There Evidence That Cruciferous Vegetables Can Help Reduce Cancer Risk In People?

Researchers have investigated possible associations between intake of cruciferous vegetables and the risk of cancer. The evidence has been reviewed by various experts. Key studies regarding four common forms of cancer are described briefly below.

- Prostate cancer: Cohort studies in the Netherlands, United States, and Europe have examined a wide range of daily cruciferous vegetable intakes and found little or no association with prostate cancer risk. However, some case-control studies have found that people who ate greater amounts of cruciferous vegetables had a lower risk of prostate cancer.

- Colorectal cancer: Cohort studies in the United States and the Netherlands have generally found no association between cruciferous vegetable intake and colorectal cancer risk. The exception is one study in the Netherlands—the Netherlands Cohort Study on Diet and Cancer—in which women (but not men) who had a high intake of cruciferous vegetables had a reduced risk of colon (but not rectal) cancer.

- Lung cancer: Cohort studies in Europe, the Netherlands, and the United States have had varying results. Most studies have reported little association, but one U.S. analysis—using data from the Nurses' Health Study and the Health Professionals' Follow-up Study—showed that women who ate more than 5 servings of cruciferous vegetables per week had a lower risk of lung cancer.

- Breast cancer: One case-control study found that women who ate greater amounts of cruciferous vegetables had a lower risk of breast cancer. A meta-analysis of studies conducted in the United States, Canada, Sweden, and the Netherlands found no association between cruciferous vegetable intake and breast cancer risk. An additional cohort study of women in the United States similarly showed only a weak association with breast cancer risk.

A few studies have shown that the bioactive components of cruciferous vegetables can have beneficial effects on biomarkers of cancer-related processes in people. For example, one study found that indole-3-carbinol was more effective than placebo in reducing the growth of abnormal cells on the surface of the cervix.

In addition, several case-control studies have shown that specific forms of the gene that encodes glutathione S-transferase, which is the enzyme that metabolizes and helps eliminate isothiocyanates from the body, may influence the association between cruciferous vegetable intake and human lung and colorectal cancer risk.

Saturated Fat, Cholesterol, And Coronary Heart Disease

When you follow a heart-healthy eating plan, you should:

- Eat less than 10 percent of your daily calories from saturated fats found naturally in foods that come from animals and some plants.

- Limit intake of *trans* fats to as low as possible by limiting foods that contain high amounts of *trans* fats.

The following are examples of foods that are high in saturated or *trans* fats.

- **Saturated fats** are found in high amounts in fatty cuts of meat, poultry with skin, whole-milk dairy foods, butter, lard, and coconut and palm oils.

- *trans* **fats** are found in high amounts in foods made with partially hydrogenated oils, such as some desserts, microwave popcorn, frozen pizza, stick margarines, and coffee creamers.

To help you limit your intake of saturated fats and *trans* fats:

- Read the nutrition labels and replace foods high in saturated fats with leaner, lower-fat animal products or vegetable oils, such as olive or canola oil instead of butter. Foods that are higher in saturated fats, such as fatty meats and high-fat dairy products, tend to be higher in dietary cholesterol that should also be limited.

- Read the nutrition labels and choose foods that do not contain *trans* fats. Some *trans* fats naturally occur in very small amounts in dairy products and meats. Foods containing these very low levels of natural *trans* fats do not need to be eliminated from your diet because they have other important nutrients.

Sodium And Hypertension

Salt And High Blood Pressure

- Research strongly shows a dose-dependent relationship between consuming too much salt and raised levels of blood pressure.

- When salt intake is reduced, blood pressure begins decreasing within weeks on average.

- Populations who consume diets low in salt do not experience the increase in blood pressure with age that is seen in most Western countries.

Is It Salt Or Is It Sodium?

- Sodium chloride is the chemical name for salt.

- The words salt and sodium are not exactly the same, yet these words are often used in place of each other. For example, the Nutrition Facts Panel uses "sodium," whereas the front of the package may say "low salt."

- Ninety percent of the sodium we consume is in the form of salt.

Reducing Sodium, Reducing Cardiovascular Disease Burden

• Even if a person does not have high blood pressure, the lower one's blood pressure in general, the lower the risk of heart disease and stroke.

• Sodium intake from processed and restaurant foods contributes to high rates of high blood pressure, heart attack, and stroke. Because nearly 400,000 deaths each year are attributed to high blood pressure, decreasing sodium intake could prevent thousands of deaths annually.

Nitrates And Cancer

There is limited evidence that nitrite may cause some cancers of the gastrointestinal tract in humans.

The International Agency for Research on Cancer (IARC) noted that the presence of nitrite and some types of amines or amides in the acid environment of the stomach may result in the production of some cancer-causing N-nitroso compounds; under these conditions, IARC determined that ingested nitrate and nitrite is probably carcinogenic to humans. The U.S. Environmental Protection Agency (EPA) has not classified nitrate or nitrite for carcinogenicity.

Chapter 51

Heart Healthy Eating

Eat For A Healthy Heart

Making healthy food choices is one important thing you can do to reduce your risk of heart disease—the leading cause of death of men and women in the United States.

According to the American Heart Association, about 80 million adults in the United States have at least one form of heart disease—disorders that prevent the heart from functioning normally—including coronary artery disease, heart rhythm problems, heart defects, infections, and cardiomyopathy (thickening or enlargement of the heart muscle).

Experts say you can reduce the risk of developing these problems with lifestyle changes that include eating a healthy diet. But with racks full of books and magazines about food and recipes, what is the best diet for a healthy heart?

U.S. Food and Drug Administration's (FDA) nutrition expert Barbara Schneeman says to follow these simple guidelines when preparing meals:

- balance calories to manage body weight

- eat at least 4.5 cups of fruits and vegetables a day, including a variety of dark-green, red, and orange vegetables, beans, and peas

- eat seafood (including oily fish) in place of some meat and poultry

- eat whole grains—the equivalent of at least three 1-ounce servings a day

About This Chapter: Information in this chapter is excerpted from "Eat for a Healthy Heart," U.S. Food and Drug Administration (FDA), July 6, 2016.

- use oils to replace solid fats

- use fat-free or low-fat versions of dairy products

The general recommendation is to eat less than 2,300 mg. of sodium a day. The government estimates that about half the U.S. population is in one of those three categories.

Packaged And Restaurant Food

Schneeman, who heads FDA's Office of Nutrition, Labeling, and Dietary Supplements, says one way to make sure you're adhering to healthy guidelines is by using the nutrition labels on the packaged foods you buy.

"Product labels give consumers the power to compare foods quickly and easily so they can judge which products best fit into a heart healthy diet or meet other dietary needs," Schneeman says. "Remember, when you see a percent DV (daily value of key nutrients) on the label, 5 percent or less is low and 20 percent or more is high."

Follow these guidelines when using processed foods or eating in restaurants:

- Choose lean meats and poultry. Bake it, broil it, or grill it.

- In a restaurant, opt for steamed, grilled, or broiled dishes instead of those that are fried or sautéed.

- Look on product labels for foods low in saturated fats, trans fats, and cholesterol. Most of the fats you eat should come from polyunsaturated and monounsaturated fats, such as those found in some types of fish, nuts, and vegetable oils.

- Check product labels for foods high in potassium (unless you've been advised to restrict the amount of potassium you eat). Potassium counteracts some of the effects of salt on blood pressure.

- Choose foods and beverages low in added sugars. Read the ingredient list to make sure that added sugars are not among the first ingredients. Ingredients in the largest amounts are listed first. Some names for added sugars include sucrose, glucose, high fructose corn syrup, corn syrup, maple syrup, and fructose. The nutrition facts on the product label give the total sugar content.

- Pick foods that provide dietary fiber, like fruits, beans, vegetables, and whole grains.

Chapter 52

The Childhood Obesity Problem

Childhood Obesity Facts

- Childhood obesity has more than doubled in children and quadrupled in adolescents in the past 30 years.

- The percentage of children aged 6–11 years in the United States who were obese increased from 7 percent in 1980 to nearly 18 percent in 2012. Similarly, the percentage of adolescents aged 12–19 years who were obese increased from 5 percent to nearly 21 percent over the same period.

- In 2012, more than one third of children and adolescents were overweight or obese.

- *Overweight* is defined as having excess body weight for a particular height from fat, muscle, bone, water, or a combination of these factors. Obesity is defined as having excess body fat.

- Overweight and obesity are the result of "caloric imbalance"—too few calories expended for the amount of calories consumed—and are affected by various genetic, behavioral, and environmental factors.

Childhood Obesity Causes

Childhood obesity is a complex health issue. It occurs when a child is well above the normal or healthy weight for his or her age and height. The main causes of excess weight in

About This Chapter: Information in this chapter is excerpted from "Childhood Obesity Facts," Centers for Disease Control and Prevention (CDC), August 27, 2015; and information from "Overweight and Obesity," Centers for Disease Control and Prevention (CDC), April 27, 2012. Reviewed September 2016.

youth are similar to those in adults, including individual causes such as behavior and genetics. Behaviors can include dietary patterns, physical activity, inactivity, medication use, and other exposures. Additional contributing factors in our society include the food and physical activity environment, education and skills, and food marketing and promotion.

Behavior

Healthy behaviors include a healthy diet pattern and regular physical activity. Energy balance of the number of calories consumed from foods and beverages with the number of calories the body uses for activity plays a role in preventing excess weight gain. A healthy diet pattern follows the *Dietary Guidelines for Americans,* which emphasizes eating whole grains, fruits, vegetables, lean protein, low-fat and fat-free dairy products and drinking water. The *Physical Activity Guidelines for Americans* recommends children do at least 60 minutes of physical activity every day.

Having a healthy diet pattern and regular physical activity is also important for long-term health benefits and prevention of chronic diseases such as type 2 diabetes and heart disease.

Community Environment

American society has become characterized by environments that promote increased consumption of less healthy food and physical inactivity. It can be difficult for children to make healthy food choices and get enough physical activity when they are exposed to environments in their home, child care center, school, or community that are influenced by—

- **Advertising of less healthy foods.**

  Nearly half of American middle and high schools allow advertising of less healthy foods, which impacts students' ability to make healthy food choices. In addition, foods high in total calories, sugars, salt, and fat, and low in nutrients are highly advertised and marketed through media targeted to children and adolescents, while advertising for healthier foods is almost nonexistent in comparison.

- **Variation in licensure regulations among child care centers.**

  More than 12 million children regularly spend time in child care arrangements outside the home. However, not all states use licensing regulations to ensure that child care facilities encourage more healthful eating and physical activity.

- **No safe and appealing place, in many communities, to play or be active.**

  Many communities are built in ways that make it difficult or unsafe to be physically active. For some families, getting to parks and recreation centers may be difficult, and public transportation may not be available. For many children, safe routes for walking or biking to school or play may not exist. Half of the children in the United States do not have a park, community center, and sidewalk in their neighborhood. Only 27 states have policies directing community-scale design.

- **Limited access to healthy affordable foods.**

Some people have less access to stores and supermarkets that sell healthy, affordable food such as fruits and vegetables, especially in rural, minority, and lower-income neighborhoods. Supermarket access is associated with a reduced risk for obesity. Choosing healthy foods is difficult for parents who live in areas with an overabundance of food retailers that tend to sell less healthy food, such as convenience stores and fast food restaurants.

- **Greater availability of high-energy-dense foods and sugar sweetened beverages.**

High-energy-dense foods are ones that have a lot of calories in each bite. A recent study among children showed that a high-energy-dense diet is associated with a higher risk for excess body fat during childhood. Sugar sweetened beverages are the largest source of added sugar and an important contributor of calories in the diets of children in the United States. High consumption of sugar sweetened beverages, which have few, if any, nutrients, has been associated with obesity. On a typical day, 80 percent of youth drink sugar sweetened beverages.

- **Increasing portion sizes.**

Portion sizes of less healthy foods and beverages have increased over time in restaurants, grocery stores, and vending machines. Research shows that children eat more without realizing it if they are served larger portions. This can mean they are consuming a lot of extra calories, especially when eating high-calorie foods.

- **Lack of breastfeeding support.**

Breastfeeding protects against childhood overweight and obesity. However, in the United States, while 75 percent of mothers start out breastfeeding, only 13 percent of babies are exclusively breastfed at the end of 6 months. The success rate among mothers who want to breastfeed can be improved through active support from their families, friends, communities, clinicians, healthcare leaders, employers, and policymakers.

Health Effects Of Childhood Obesity

Childhood obesity has both immediate and long-term effects on health and well-being.

Immediate health effects:

- Obese youth are more likely to have risk factors for cardiovascular disease, such as high cholesterol or high blood pressure. In a population-based sample of 5- to 17-year-olds, 70 percent of obese youth had at least one risk factor for cardiovascular disease.

- Obese adolescents are more likely to have prediabetes, a condition in which blood glucose levels indicate a high risk for development of diabetes.

- Children and adolescents who are obese are at greater risk for bone and joint problems, sleep apnea, and social and psychological problems such as stigmatization and poor self-esteem.

Long-term health effects:

- Children and adolescents who are obese are likely to be obese as adults 11–14 and are therefore more at risk for adult health problems such as heart disease, type 2 diabetes, stroke, several types of cancer, and osteoarthritis. One study showed that children who became obese as early as age 2 were more likely to be obese as adults.

- Overweight and obesity are associated with increased risk for many types of cancer, including cancer of the breast, colon, endometrium, esophagus, kidney, pancreas, gall bladder, thyroid, ovary, cervix, and prostate, as well as multiple myeloma and Hodgkin lymphoma.

Prevention

- Healthy lifestyle habits, including healthy eating and physical activity, can lower the risk of becoming obese and developing related diseases.

- The dietary and physical activity behaviors of children and adolescents are influenced by many sectors of society, including families, communities, schools, child care settings, medical care providers, faith-based institutions, government agencies, the media, and the food and beverage industries and entertainment industries.

- Schools play a particularly critical role by establishing a safe and supportive environment with policies and practices that support healthy behaviors. Schools also provide opportunities for students to learn about and practice healthy eating and physical activity behaviors.

Consequences Of Obesity

Health Risks Now

- Obesity during childhood can have a harmful effect on the body in a variety of ways. Children who are obese have a greater risk of—
  - High blood pressure and high cholesterol, which are risk factors for cardiovascular disease (CVD). In one study, 70 percent of obese children had at least one CVD risk factor, and 39 percent had two or more.
  - Increased risk of impaired glucose tolerance, insulin resistance and type 2 diabetes.
  - Breathing problems, such as sleep apnea, and asthma.
  - Joint problems and musculoskeletal discomfort.
  - Fatty liver disease, gallstones, and gastro-esophageal reflux (i.e., heartburn).
  - Psychological stress such as depression, behavioral problems, and issues in school.
  - Low self-esteem and low self-reported quality of life.
  - Impaired social, physical, and emotional functioning.

Health Risks Later

- Children who are obese are more likely to become obese adults. Adult obesity is associated with a number of serious health conditions including heart disease, diabetes, metabolic syndrome, and cancer.
- If children are obese, obesity and disease risk factors in adulthood are likely to be more severe.

Chapter 53

Dealing With Celiac Disease

What Is Celiac Disease?

Celiac disease is a digestive disorder that damages the small intestine. The disease is triggered by eating foods containing gluten. Gluten is a protein found naturally in wheat, barley, and rye, and is common in foods such as bread, pasta, cookies, and cakes. Many pre-packaged foods, lip balms and lipsticks, hair and skin products, toothpastes, vitamin and nutrient supplements, and, rarely, medicines, contain gluten.

> Celiac disease can be very serious. The disease can cause long-lasting digestive problems and keep your body from getting all the nutrients it needs. Celiac disease can also affect the body outside the intestine.

Celiac disease is different from gluten sensitivity or wheat intolerance. If you have gluten sensitivity, you may have symptoms similar to those of celiac disease, such as abdominal pain and tiredness. Unlike celiac disease, gluten sensitivity does not damage the small intestine.

Celiac disease is also different from a wheat allergy. In both cases, your body's immune system reacts to wheat. However, some symptoms in wheat allergies, such as having itchy eyes or a hard time breathing, are different from celiac disease. Wheat allergies also do not cause long-term damage to the small intestine.

About This Chapter: Information in this chapter is excerpted from "Celiac Disease," National Institute of Diabetes and Digestive and Kidney Diseases (NIDDK), June 16, 2016.

What Are The Complications Of Celiac Disease?

Long-term complications of celiac disease include:

- malnutrition, a condition in which you don't get enough vitamins, minerals, and other nutrients you need to be healthy

- accelerated osteoporosis or bone softening, known as osteomalacia

- nervous system problems

- problems related to reproduction

Rare complications can include:

- intestinal cancer

- liver diseases

- lymphoma, a cancer of part of the immune system called the lymph system that includes the gut

> In rare cases, you may continue to have trouble absorbing nutrients even though you have been following a strict gluten-free diet. If you have this condition, called refractory celiac disease, your intestines are severely damaged and can't heal. You may need to receive nutrients through an IV.

How Do Doctors Treat Celiac Disease?

A Gluten-Free Diet

Doctors treat celiac disease with a gluten-free diet. Gluten is a protein found naturally in wheat, barley, and rye that triggers a reaction if you have celiac disease. Symptoms greatly improve for most people with celiac disease who stick to a gluten-free diet. In recent years, grocery stores and restaurants have added many more gluten-free foods and products, making it easier to stay gluten free.

Your doctor may refer you to a dietitian who specializes in treating people with celiac disease. The dietitian will teach you how to avoid gluten while following a healthy diet. He or she will help you

- check food and product labels for gluten

- design everyday meal plans

- make healthy choices about the types of foods to eat

For most people, following a gluten-free diet will heal damage in the small intestine and prevent more damage. You may see symptoms improve within days to weeks of starting the diet. The small intestine usually heals in 3 to 6 months in children. Complete healing can take several years in adults. Once the intestine heals, the villi, which were damaged by the disease, regrow and will absorb nutrients from food into the bloodstream normally.

Gluten-Free Diet And Dermatitis Herpetiformis

If you have dermatitis herpetiformis—an itchy, blistering skin rash—skin symptoms generally respond to a gluten-free diet. However, skin symptoms may return if you add gluten back into your diet. Medicines such as dapsone, taken by mouth, can control the skin symptoms. People who take dapsone need to have regular blood tests to check for side effects from the medicine.

Dapsone does not treat intestinal symptoms or damage, which is why you should stay on a gluten-free diet if you have the rash. Even when you follow a gluten-free diet, the rash may take months or even years to fully heal—and often comes back over the years.

Avoiding Medicines And Nonfood Products That May Contain Gluten

In addition to prescribing a gluten-free diet, your doctor will want you to avoid all hidden sources of gluten. If you have celiac disease, ask a pharmacist about ingredients in

- herbal and nutritional supplements

- prescription and over-the-counter medicines

- vitamin and mineral supplements

You also could take in or transfer from your hands to your mouth other products that contain gluten without knowing it. Products that may contain gluten include

- children's modeling dough, such as Play-Doh

- cosmetics

- lipstick, lip gloss, and lip balm

- skin and hair products

- toothpaste and mouthwash

- communion wafers

Medications are rare sources of gluten. Even if gluten is present in a medicine, it is likely to be in such small quantities that it would not cause any symptoms.

> Reading product labels can sometimes help you avoid gluten. Some product makers label their products as being gluten-free. If a product label doesn't list the product's ingredients, ask the maker of the product for an ingredients list.

What If Changing To A Gluten-Free Diet Isn't Working?

If you don't improve after starting a gluten-free diet, you may still be eating or using small amounts of gluten. You probably will start responding to the gluten-free diet once you find and cut out all hidden sources of gluten. Hidden sources of gluten include additives made with wheat, such as

- modified food starch

- malt flavoring

- preservatives

- stabilizers

If you still have symptoms even after changing your diet, you may have other conditions or disorders that are more common with celiac disease, such as irritable bowel syndrome (IBS), lactose intolerance, microscopic colitis, dysfunction of the pancreas, and small intestinal bacterial overgrowth.

What Should I Avoid Eating If I Have Celiac Disease?

Avoiding foods with gluten, a protein found naturally in wheat, rye, and barley, is critical in treating celiac disease. Removing gluten from your diet will improve symptoms, heal damage to your small intestine, and prevent further damage over time. While you may need to avoid certain foods, the good news is that many healthy, gluten-free foods and products are available.

You should avoid all products that contain gluten, such as most cereal, grains, and pasta, and many processed foods. Be sure to always read food ingredient lists carefully to make sure the food you want to eat doesn't have gluten. In addition, discuss gluten-free food choices with a dietitian or healthcare professional who specializes in celiac disease.

What Should I Eat If I Have Celiac Disease?

Foods such as meat, fish, fruits, vegetables, rice, and potatoes without additives or seasonings do not contain gluten and are part of a well-balanced diet. You can eat gluten-free types of bread, pasta, and other foods that are now easier to find in stores, restaurants, and at special food companies. You also can eat potato, rice, soy, amaranth, quinoa, buckwheat, or bean flour instead of wheat flour.

In the past, doctors and dietitians advised against eating oats if you have celiac disease. Evidence suggests that most people with the disease can safely eat moderate amounts of oats, as long as they did not come in contact with wheat gluten during processing. You should talk with your healthcare team about whether to include oats in your diet.

When shopping and eating out, remember to

- Read food labels—especially on canned, frozen, and processed foods—for ingredients that contain gluten.

- Identify foods labelled "gluten-free;" by law, these foods must contain less than 20 parts per million, well below the threshold to cause problems in the great majority of patients with celiac disease.

- Ask restaurant servers and chefs about how they prepare the food and what is in it.

- Find out whether a gluten-free menu is available.

- Ask a dinner or party host about gluten-free options before attending a social gathering.

Foods labeled gluten-free tend to cost more than the same foods that have gluten. You may find that naturally gluten-free foods are less expensive. With practice, looking for gluten can become second nature.

Is A Gluten-Free Diet Safe If I Don't Have Celiac Disease?

In recent years, more people without celiac disease have adopted a gluten-free diet, believing that avoiding gluten is healthier or could help them lose weight. No current data suggests that the general public should maintain a gluten-free diet for weight loss or better health.

A gluten-free diet isn't always a healthy diet. For instance, a gluten-free diet may not provide enough of the nutrients, vitamins, and minerals the body needs, such as fiber, iron, and calcium. Some gluten-free products can be high in calories and sugar.

If you think you might have celiac disease, don't start avoiding gluten without first speaking with your doctor. If your doctor diagnoses you with celiac disease, he or she will put you on a gluten-free diet.

Chapter 54
Dealing With Diabetes

Learn About Diabetes

Diabetes means that your blood glucose (blood sugar) is too high. There are two main types of diabetes.

Type 1 diabetes - the body does not make insulin. Insulin helps the body use glucose from food for energy. People with type 1 need to take insulin every day.

Type 2 diabetes - the body does not make or use insulin well. People with type 2 often need to take pills or insulin. Type 2 is the most common form of diabetes.

Diabetes: Diet And Eating

You can take good care of yourself and your diabetes by learning

- what to eat

- how much to eat

- when to eat

Making wise food choices can help you

- feel good every day

- lose weight if you need to

- lower your risk for heart disease, stroke, and other problems caused by diabetes

About This Chapter: Information in this chapter is excerpted from "Step 1: Learn about Diabetes," National Institute of Diabetes and Digestive and Kidney Diseases (NIDDK), December 15, 2015; and information from "Diabetes Diet and Eating," National Institute of Diabetes and Digestive and Kidney Diseases (NIDDK), June 2014.

Healthful eating helps keep your blood glucose, also called blood sugar, in your target range. Physical activity and, if needed, diabetes medicines also help. The diabetes target range is the blood glucose level suggested by diabetes experts for good health. You can help prevent health problems by keeping your blood glucose levels on target.

Blood Glucose Levels

What Should My Blood Glucose Levels Be?

Table 54.1. Target Blood Glucose Levels

Target Blood Glucose Levels For People With Diabetes	
Before meals	70 to 130
1 to 2 hours after the start of a meal	less than 180

Ask your doctor how often you should check your blood glucose on your own. Also ask your doctor for an A1C test at least twice a year. Your A1C number gives your average blood glucose for the past 3 months. The results from your blood glucose checks and your A1C test will tell you whether your diabetes care plan is working.

How Can I Keep My Blood Glucose Levels On Target?

You can keep your blood glucose levels on target by

- making wise food choices

- being physically active

- taking medicines if needed

For people taking certain diabetes medicines, following a schedule for meals, snacks, and physical activity is best. However, some diabetes medicines allow for more flexibility. You'll work with your healthcare team to create a diabetes plan that's best for you.

Talk with your doctor or diabetes teacher about how many meals and snacks to eat each day.

Your Diabetes Medicines

What you eat and when you eat affect how your diabetes medicines work. Talk with your doctor or diabetes teacher about when to take your diabetes medicines.

Your Physical Activity Plan

What you eat and when also depend on how much you exercise. Physical activity is an important part of staying healthy and controlling your blood glucose. Keep these points in mind:

- Talk with your doctor about what types of exercise are safe for you.

- Make sure your shoes fit well and your socks stay clean and dry. Check your feet for redness or sores after exercising. Call your doctor if you have sores that do not heal.

- Warm up and stretch for 5 to 10 minutes before you exercise. Then cool down for several minutes after you exercise. For example, walk slowly at first, stretch, and then walk faster. Finish up by walking slowly again.

- Ask your doctor whether you should exercise if your blood glucose level is high.

- Ask your doctor whether you should have a snack before you exercise.

- Know the signs of low blood glucose, also called hypoglycemia. Always carry food or glucose tablets to treat low blood glucose.

- Always wear your medical identification or other ID.

- Find an exercise buddy. Many people find they are more likely to do something active if a friend joins them.

Low Blood Glucose (Hypoglycemia)

Low blood glucose can make you feel shaky, weak, confused, irritable, hungry, or tired. You may sweat a lot or get a headache. If you have these symptoms, check your blood glucose. If it is below 70, have one of the following right away:

- 3 or 4 glucose tablets

- 1 serving of glucose gel-the amount equal to 15 grams of carbohydrate

- 1/2 cup (4 ounces) of any fruit juice

- 1/2 cup (4 ounces) of a regular **(not diet)** soft drink

- 1 cup (8 ounces) of milk

- 5 or 6 pieces of hard candy

- 1 tablespoon of sugar or honey

After 15 minutes, check your blood glucose again. If it's still too low, have another serving. Repeat these steps until your blood glucose level is 70 or higher. If it will be an hour or more before your next meal, have a snack as well.

The Diabetes Food Pyramid

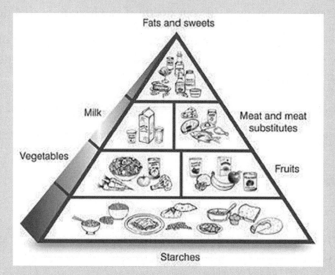

Figure 54.1. Food Pyramid

The diabetes food pyramid can help you make wise food choices. It divides foods into groups, based on what they contain. Eat more from the groups at the bottom of the pyramid, and less from the groups at the top. Foods from the starches, fruits, vegetables, and milk groups are highest in carbohydrate. They affect your blood glucose levels the most.

How Much Should I Eat Each Day?

Talk with your diabetes teacher about how to make a meal plan that fits the way you usually eat, your daily routine, and your diabetes medicines. Then make your own plan.

Starches

Starches are bread, grains, cereal, pasta, and starchy vegetables like corn and potatoes. They provide carbohydrate, vitamins, minerals, and fiber. Whole grain starches are healthier because they have more vitamins, minerals, and fiber.

Eat some starches at each meal. Eating starches is healthy for everyone, including people with diabetes.

Examples of starches are:

- Beans
- Bread
- Cereal
- Corn
- Crackers
- Lentils

- Pasta
- Potatoes
- Pretzels
- Rice
- Tortillas
- Yams

What Are Healthy Ways To Eat Starches

- Buy whole grain breads and cereals.

- Eat fewer fried and high-fat starches such as regular tortilla chips and potato chips, french fries, pastries, or biscuits. Try pretzels, fat-free popcorn, baked tortilla chips or potato chips, baked potatoes, or low-fat muffins.

- Use low-fat or fat-free plain yogurt or fat-free sour cream instead of regular sour cream on a baked potato.

- Use mustard instead of mayonnaise on a sandwich.

- Use low-fat or fat-free substitutes such as low-fat mayonnaise or light margarine on bread, rolls, or toast.

- Eat cereal with fat-free (skim) or low-fat (1%) milk.

Vegetables

Vegetables provide vitamins, minerals, and fiber. They are low in carbohydrate.

Examples of vegetables are:

- Broccoli
- Cabbage
- Carrots
- Celery

- Chilies
- Green beans
- Greens
- Lettuce

- Peppers
- Spinach
- Tomatoes
- Vegetable juice

What Are Healthy Ways To Eat Vegetables?

- Eat raw and cooked vegetables with little or no fat, sauces, or dressings.

- Try low-fat or fat-free salad dressing on raw vegetables or salads.

- Steam vegetables using water or low-fat broth.

- Mix in some chopped onion or garlic.

- Use a little vinegar or some lemon or lime juice.

- Add a small piece of lean ham or smoked turkey instead of fat to vegetables when cooking.

- Sprinkle with herbs and spices.

- If you do use a small amount of fat, use canola oil, olive oil, or soft margarines (liquid or tub types) instead of fat from meat, butter, or shortening.

Fruits

Fruits provide carbohydrate, vitamins, minerals, and fiber.

Examples of fruits include:

- Apples
- Bananas
- Berries
- Canned fruit
- Dried fruit
- Fruit juice
- Grapefruit
- Guava
- Mango
- Oranges
- Papaya
- Peaches
- Raisins
- Strawberries
- Watermelon

What Are Healthy Ways To Eat Fruits?

- Eat fruits raw or cooked, as juice with no sugar added, canned in their own juice, or dried.

- Buy smaller pieces of fruit.

- Choose pieces of fruit more often than fruit juice. Whole fruit is more filling and has more fiber.

- Save high-sugar and high-fat fruit desserts such as peach cobbler or cherry pie for special occasions.

Milk

Milk provides carbohydrate, protein, calcium, vitamins, and minerals.

What Are Healthy Ways To Have Milk?

- Drink fat-free (skim) or low-fat (1%) milk.

- Eat low-fat or fat-free fruit yogurt sweetened with a low-calorie sweetener.

- Use low-fat plain yogurt as a substitute for sour cream.

Meat And Meat Substitutes

The meat and meat substitutes group includes meat, poultry, eggs, cheese, fish, and tofu. Eat small amounts of some of these foods each day.

Meat and meat substitutes provide protein, vitamins, and minerals.

Examples of meat and meat substitutes include:

- Beef
- Canned tuna or other fish
- Cheese
- Chicken
- Cottage cheese
- Eggs
- Fish
- Lamb
- Peanut butter
- Pork
- Tofu
- Turkey

What Are Healthy Ways To Eat Meat And Meat Substitutes?

- Buy cuts of beef, pork, ham, and lamb that have only a little fat on them. Trim off the extra fat.

- Eat chicken or turkey without the skin.

- Cook meat and meat substitutes in low-fat ways:

  - broil
  - grill
  - stir-fry
  - roast
  - steam
  - microwave

- To add more flavor, use vinegars, lemon juice, soy sauce, salsa, ketchup, barbecue sauce, herbs, and spices.

- Cook eggs using cooking spray or a non-stick pan.

- Limit the amount of nuts, peanut butter, and fried foods you eat. They are high in fat.

- Check food labels. Choose low-fat or fat-free cheese.

Fats And Sweets

Limit the amount of fats and sweets you eat. Fats and sweets are not as nutritious as other foods. Fats have a lot of calories. Sweets can be high in carbohydrate and fat. Some contain saturated fats, trans fats, and cholesterol that increase your risk of heart disease. Limiting these foods will help you lose weight and keep your blood glucose and blood fats under control.

Examples of fats include:

- Avocado
- Bacon
- Butter
- Cream cheese
- Margarine
- Mayonnaise
- Oil
- Olives
- Salad dressing

Examples of sweets include:

- Cake
- Cookies
- Doughnuts
- Ice cream
- Pie
- Syrup

How Can I Satisfy My Sweet Tooth?

Try having sugar-free popsicles, diet soda, fat-free ice cream or frozen yogurt, or sugar-free hot cocoa mix.

Other tips:

- Share desserts in restaurants.

- Order small or child-size servings of ice cream or frozen yogurt.

- Divide homemade desserts into small servings and wrap each individually. Freeze extra servings.

Remember, fat-free and low-sugar foods still have calories. Talk with your diabetes teacher about how to fit sweets into your meal plan.

> ## Alcoholic Drinks
> Alcoholic drinks have calories but no nutrients. If you have alcoholic drinks on an empty stomach, they can make your blood glucose level go too low. Alcoholic drinks also can raise your blood fats. If you want to have alcoholic drinks, talk with your doctor or diabetes teacher about how much to have.

Your Meal Plan

Plan your meals and snacks for one day. Work with your diabetes teacher if you need help.

Measuring Your Food

To make sure your food servings are the right size, you can use

- measuring cups

- measuring spoons

- a food scale

The Nutrition Facts label on food packages tells you how much of that food is in one serving.

When You're Sick

Take care of yourself when you're sick. Being sick can make your blood glucose go too high. Tips on what to do include the following:

- Check your blood glucose level every 4 hours. Write down the results.

- Keep taking your diabetes medicines. You need them even if you can't keep food down.

- Drink at least one cup (8 ounces) of water or other calorie-free, caffeine-free liquid every hour while you're awake.

- If you can't eat your usual food, try drinking juice or eating crackers, popsicles, or soup.

- If you can't eat at all, drink clear liquids such as ginger ale. Eat or drink something with sugar in it if you have trouble keeping food down, because you still need calories. If you can't eat enough, you increase your risk of low blood glucose, also called hypoglycemia.

- In people with type 1 diabetes, when blood glucose is high, the body produces ketones. Ketones can make you sick. Test your urine or blood for ketones if

  - your blood glucose is above 240

  - you can't keep food or liquids down

- Call your healthcare provider right away if

  - your blood glucose has been above 240 for longer than a day

  - you have ketones

  - you feel sleepier than usual

  - you have trouble breathing

  - you can't think clearly

  - you throw up more than once

  - you've had diarrhea for more than 6 hours

Chapter 55

Dealing With Food Allergies

Prevention

There is currently no cure for food allergies. You can only prevent the symptoms of food allergy by avoiding the allergenic food. After you and your healthcare professional have identified the food(s) to which you are sensitive, you must remove them from your diet.

Read Food Labels

You must read the list of ingredients on the label of each prepared food that you are considering eating. Many allergens, such as peanut, egg, and milk, appear in prepared foods you normally would not associate with those foods.

Since 2006, the U.S. food manufacturers have been required by law to list the ingredients of prepared foods. In addition, food manufacturers must use plain language to disclose whether their products contain any of the top eight allergenic foods—egg, milk, peanut, tree nuts, soy, wheat, shellfish, and fish. Be aware that some labels say "may contain."

Keep Clean

Simple measures of cleanliness can remove most allergens from the environment of a person with food allergy. For example, simply washing your hands with soap and water will remove peanut allergens, and most household cleaners will remove allergens from surfaces.

About This Chapter: Information in this chapter is excerpted from "Food Allergy: An Overview," National Institute of Allergy and Infectious Diseases (NIAID), July 2012. Reviewed September 2016.

Treatment Of A Food Allergy Reaction

Unintentional Exposure

When you have food allergies, you must be prepared to treat an unintentional exposure. Talk to your healthcare professional and develop a plan to protect yourself in case of an unintentional exposure to the food. For example, you should

- wear a medical alert bracelet or necklace

- carry an auto-injector device containing **epinephrine** (adrenaline)

Mild Symptoms

Talk to your healthcare professional to find out what medicines may relieve mild food allergy symptoms that are *not part of an anaphylactic reaction*. However, be aware that it is very hard for you to know which reactions are mild and which may lead to anaphylaxis.

Exercise-Induced Food Allergy

Exercise-induced food allergy is a rare situation that requires more than simply eating food to start a reaction. This type of reaction occurs after someone eats a specific food before exercising. As exercise increases and body temperature rises

- itching and light-headedness start
- hives may appear
- anaphylaxis may develop

Treating exercised-induced food allergy is simple—avoid eating for a couple of hours before exercising.

Crustacean shellfish, alcohol, tomatoes, cheese, and celery are common causes of exercise-induced food allergy reactions.

Chapter 56
Dealing With Lactose Intolerance

What Is Lactose?

Lactose is a sugar found in milk and milk products. The small intestine produces lactase, an enzyme that breaks down lactose. The small intestine is an organ that breaks down the food you eat. Enzymes are proteins that help to cause chemical changes in the body.

What Is Lactose Intolerance?

Lactose intolerance means you have symptoms such as bloating, diarrhea, and gas after you have milk or milk products.

If your small intestine does not produce much lactase, you cannot break down much lactose. Lactose that does not break down goes to your colon. The colon is an organ that absorbs water from stool and changes it from a liquid to a solid form. In your colon, bacteria that normally live in the colon break down the lactose and create fluid and gas, causing you to have symptoms.

The causes of low lactase in your small intestine can include the following:

- In some people, the small intestine makes less lactase starting at about age 2, which may lead to symptoms of lactose intolerance. Other people start to have symptoms later, when they are teenagers or adults.

- Infection, disease, or other problems that harm the small intestine can cause low lactase levels. Low lactase levels can cause you to become lactose intolerant until your small intestine heals.

About This Chapter: Information in this chapter is excerpted from "Lactose Intolerance," National Institute of Diabetes and Digestive and Kidney Diseases (NIDDK), June 2014.

Not all people with low lactase levels have symptoms. If you have symptoms, you are lactose intolerant.

Most people who are lactose intolerant can have some milk or milk products and not have symptoms. The amount of lactose that causes symptoms is different from person to person.

People sometimes confuse lactose intolerance with a milk allergy. While lactose intolerance is a digestive problem, a milk allergy is a reaction by the body's immune system to one or more milk proteins. If you have a milk allergy, having even a small amount of milk or milk product can be life threatening. A milk allergy most commonly occurs in the first year of life. Lactose intolerance occurs more often during the teen years or adulthood.

Can Anyone Have Lactose Intolerance?

Anyone can have lactose intolerance. In the United States, some people are more likely to be lactose intolerant, including

- African Americans

- American Indians

- Hispanics/Latinos

- Asian Americans

People with European heritage are least likely to be lactose intolerant.

What Are The Symptoms Of Lactose Intolerance?

Common symptoms of lactose intolerance include

- bloating, a feeling of fullness or swelling, in your belly

- pain in your belly

- diarrhea

- gas

- nausea

You may feel symptoms 30 minutes to 2 hours after you have milk or milk products. You may have mild or severe symptoms.

How Does Lactose Intolerance Affect My Health?

In addition to having unpleasant symptoms, you may have trouble getting enough nutrients, such as calcium and vitamin D. Milk and milk products are sources of calcium. Calcium is a mineral the body needs for strong bones and teeth. If you do not get enough calcium, over time your bones may become less dense and break easily.

How Does My Doctor Know If I Have Lactose Intolerance?

Your doctor will try to find out if you have lactose intolerance with the following:

- **Medical, family, and diet history.** Your doctor will ask you questions about your medical and family history, your diet, and your symptoms.

- **Physical exam.** A physical exam may help your doctor find out if you have lactose intolerance or another problem. During a physical exam, your doctor usually

  - checks for bloating in your belly

  - uses a stethoscope to listen to sounds within your belly

  - taps on your belly to check for tenderness or pain

After taking a history and completing a physical exam, your doctor may ask you to stop having milk and milk products to see if your symptoms go away. If your symptoms do not go away, your doctor might order the following tests:

- **Hydrogen breath test.** This test checks the amount of a gas called hydrogen in your breath. Normally, a person's breath only has a small amount of hydrogen after you eat lactose and the body breaks it down. Lactose that the body does not break down causes high amounts of hydrogen in the breath. For this test, you have a drink with a known amount of lactose. A doctor asks you to breathe into a balloon-type container that measures hydrogen. A doctor usually performs this test at a hospital, on an outpatient basis. Smoking and some foods and medicines may affect the results. Your doctor will tell you what foods and medicines you need to avoid before the test.

- **Stool acidity test.** If your body does not break down lactose, the lactose creates acid. The stool acidity test measures the amount of acid in the stool from a bowel movement. Doctors sometimes use this test for infants and young children. The doctor will give you a container to take home for catching and storing your child's stool. You will need to return the sample to the doctor, and the doctor will send it to a lab for testing.

How Much Lactose Can I Have?

Most people with lactose intolerance can eat or drink some lactose without symptoms. Different people can have different amounts of lactose. For example, one person may have severe symptoms after drinking a small amount of milk. Another person can drink a large amount without symptoms. Some people can easily eat yogurt and hard cheeses such as cheddar and Swiss, while other milk products cause them to have symptoms.

Research suggests that many people could have the amount of lactose in 1 cup of milk in one sitting without symptoms or with only minor symptoms. You may be able to have more lactose if you have it with meals or in small amounts throughout the day.

Many people who have lactose intolerance do not need to avoid milk or milk products completely. If you avoid milk and milk products altogether, you may take in less calcium and vitamin D than you need.

What Can I Do If I Have Lactose Intolerance?

If you have lactose intolerance, you can make changes to what you eat and drink. Some people may only need to have less lactose. Others may need to avoid lactose altogether. Using products that contain lactase helps some people.

Eating, Diet, And Nutrition

Talk with your doctor about your dietary plan. A dietary plan can help you manage the symptoms of lactose intolerance and get enough nutrients. If you have a child with lactose intolerance, follow the diet plan that your child's doctor recommends.

Milk and milk products. You may be able to have milk and milk products without symptoms if you

- drink small amounts of milk—half a cup or less—at a time
- drink small amounts of milk with meals, such as having milk with cereal or having cheese with crackers
- add small amounts of milk and milk products to your diet a little at a time and see how you feel
- eat milk products that are easier for people with lactose intolerance to break down:
  - yogurt
  - hard cheeses such as cheddar and Swiss

Lactose-free and lactose-reduced milk and milk products. You can find lactose-free and lactose-reduced milk and milk products at the grocery store. These products are just as healthy for you as regular milk and milk products.

Lactase products. You can use lactase tablets and drops when you have milk and milk products. The lactase enzyme breaks down the lactose in food. Using lactase tablets or drops can help you prevent symptoms of lactose intolerance. Check with your doctor before using these products. Some people, such as young children and pregnant and breastfeeding women, may not be able to use these products.

Calcium and Vitamin D

If you are lactose intolerant, make sure you get enough calcium each day. Milk and milk products are the most common sources of calcium. Other foods that contain calcium include

- fish with soft bones, such as canned salmon or sardines
- broccoli and other leafy green vegetables
- oranges
- almonds, Brazil nuts, and dried beans
- tofu
- products with the label showing added calcium, such as cereals, fruit juices, and soy milk

Vitamin D helps the body absorb and use calcium. Be sure to eat foods that contain vitamin D, such as eggs, liver, and certain kinds of fish, such as salmon. Also, being outside in the sunlight helps your body make vitamin D. Some companies add vitamin D to milk and milk products. If you are able to drink small amounts of milk or eat yogurt, choose those that have vitamin D added.

Talk with your doctor about how to get enough nutrients—including calcium and vitamin D—in your diet or your child's diet. Ask if you should also take a supplement to get enough calcium and vitamin D.

For safety reasons, talk with your doctor before using dietary supplements or any other non-mainstream medicine together with or in place of the treatment your doctor prescribes.

How Will I Know If A Food Or Medicine Has Lactose?

Lactose is in many food products and in some medicines.

Food Products

Lactose is in milk and all foods made with milk, such as

- ice cream

- cream

- butter

- cheese

- cottage cheese

- yogurt

Rarely, people with lactose intolerance are even bothered by small amounts of lactose. Some boxed, canned, frozen, packaged, and prepared foods contain small amounts of lactose. These foods include

- bread and other baked goods

- waffles, pancakes, biscuits, and cookies, and the mixes to make them

- prepared or frozen breakfast foods such as doughnuts, frozen waffles and pancakes, toaster pastries, and sweet rolls

- boxed breakfast cereals

- instant potatoes, soups, and breakfast drinks

- potato chips, corn chips, and other packaged snacks

- prepared meats, such as bacon, sausage, hot dogs, and lunch meats

- margarine

- salad dressings

- liquid and powdered milk-based meal replacements

- protein powders and bars

- candies

- nondairy liquid and powdered coffee creamers

- nondairy whipped toppings

Look for certain words on food labels. These words mean the food has lactose:

- milk

- lactose

- whey

- curds

- milk by-products

- nonfat dry milk powder

- dry milk solids—another name for dry milk powder

Medicines

Some medicines contain lactose, including

- prescription (OTC) medicines, such as birth control pills

- over-the-counter medicines, such as products to treat stomach acid and gas

These medicines most often cause symptoms in people with severe lactose intolerance. If you have lactose intolerance, ask your doctor if your medicines contain lactose.

Chapter 57
Understanding Foodborne Illness

What Are Foodborne Illnesses?

Foodborne illnesses are infections or irritations of the gastrointestinal (GI) tract caused by food or beverages that contain harmful bacteria, parasites, viruses, or chemicals. The GI tract is a series of hollow organs joined in a long, twisting tube from the mouth to the anus. Common symptoms of foodborne illnesses include vomiting, diarrhea, abdominal pain, fever, and chills.

Most foodborne illnesses are acute, meaning they happen suddenly and last a short time, and most people recover on their own without treatment. Rarely, foodborne illnesses may lead to more serious complications. Each year, an estimated 48 million people in the United States experience a foodborne illness. Foodborne illnesses cause about 3,000 deaths in the United States annually.

What Causes Foodborne Illnesses?

The majority of foodborne illnesses are caused by harmful bacteria and viruses. Some parasites and chemicals also cause foodborne illnesses.

Bacteria

Bacteria are tiny organisms that can cause infections of the GI tract. Not all bacteria are harmful to humans.

Some harmful bacteria may already be present in foods when they are purchased. Raw foods including meat, poultry, fish and shellfish, eggs, unpasteurized milk and dairy products,

About This Chapter: Information in this chapter is excerpted from "Foodborne Illnesses," National Institute of Diabetes and Digestive and Kidney Diseases (NIDDK), June 2014.

and fresh produce often contain bacteria that cause foodborne illnesses. Bacteria can contaminate food—making it harmful to eat—at any time during growth, harvesting or slaughter, processing, storage, and shipping.

Foods may also be contaminated with bacteria during food preparation in a restaurant or home kitchen. If food preparers do not thoroughly wash their hands, kitchen utensils, cutting boards, and other kitchen surfaces that come into contact with raw foods, cross-contamination—the spread of bacteria from contaminated food to uncontaminated food—may occur.

If hot food is not kept hot enough or cold food is not kept cold enough, bacteria may multiply. Bacteria multiply quickly when the temperature of food is between 40 and 140 degrees. Cold food should be kept below 40 degrees and hot food should be kept above 140 degrees. Bacteria multiply more slowly when food is refrigerated, and freezing food can further slow or even stop the spread of bacteria. However, bacteria in refrigerated or frozen foods become active again when food is brought to room temperature. Thoroughly cooking food kills bacteria.

Many types of bacteria cause foodborne illnesses. Examples include

- *Salmonella*, a bacterium found in many foods, including raw and undercooked meat, poultry, dairy products, and seafood. *Salmonella* may also be present on egg shells and inside eggs.

- *Campylobacter jejuni (C. jejuni)*, found in raw or undercooked chicken and unpasteurized milk.

- *Shigella*, a bacterium spread from person to person. These bacteria are present in the stools of people who are infected. If people who are infected do not wash their hands thoroughly after using the bathroom, they can contaminate food that they handle or prepare. Water contaminated with infected stools can also contaminate produce in the field.

- *Escherichia coli (E. coli)*, which includes several different strains, only a few of which cause illness in humans. *E. coli O157:H7* is the strain that causes the most severe illness. Common sources of *E. coli* include raw or undercooked hamburger, unpasteurized fruit juices and milk, and fresh produce.

- *Listeria monocytogenes (L. monocytogenes)*, which has been found in raw and undercooked meats, unpasteurized milk, soft cheeses, and ready-to-eat deli meats and hot dogs.

- *Vibrio*, a bacterium that may contaminate fish or shellfish.

- *Clostridium botulinum (C. botulinum),* a bacterium that may contaminate improperly canned foods and smoked and salted fish.

Viruses

Viruses are tiny capsules, much smaller than bacteria, that contain genetic material. Viruses cause infections that can lead to sickness. People can pass viruses to each other. Viruses are present in the stool or vomit of people who are infected. People who are infected with a virus may contaminate food and drinks, especially if they do not wash their hands thoroughly after using the bathroom.

Common sources of foodborne viruses include

- food prepared by a person infected with a virus

- shellfish from contaminated water

- produce irrigated with contaminated water

Common foodborne viruses include

- norovirus, which causes inflammation of the stomach and intestines

- hepatitis A, which causes inflammation of the liver

Parasites

Parasites are tiny organisms that live inside another organism. In developed countries such as the United States, parasitic infections are relatively rare.

Cryptosporidium parvum and *Giardia intestinalis* are parasites that are spread through water contaminated with the stools of people or animals who are infected. Foods that come into contact with contaminated water during growth or preparation can become contaminated with these parasites. Food preparers who are infected with these parasites can also contaminate foods if they do not thoroughly wash their hands after using the bathroom and before handling food.

Trichinella spiralis is a type of roundworm parasite. People may be infected with this parasite by consuming raw or undercooked pork or wild game.

Chemicals

Harmful chemicals that cause illness may contaminate foods such as

- fish or shellfish, which may feed on algae that produce toxins, leading to high concentrations of toxins in their bodies. Some types of fish, including tuna and mahi mahi, may be

317

contaminated with bacteria that produce toxins if the fish are not properly refrigerated before they are cooked or served.

- certain types of wild mushrooms.

- unwashed fruits and vegetables that contain high concentrations of pesticides.

Who Gets Foodborne Illnesses?

Anyone can get a foodborne illness. However, some people are more likely to develop foodborne illnesses than others, including

- infants and children

- pregnant women and their fetuses

- older adults

- people with weak immune systems

These groups also have a greater risk of developing severe symptoms or complications of foodborne illnesses.

What Are The Symptoms Of Foodborne Illnesses?

Symptoms of foodborne illnesses depend on the cause. Common symptoms of many foodborne illnesses include

- vomiting

- diarrhea or bloody diarrhea

- abdominal pain

- fever

- chills

Symptoms can range from mild to serious and can last from a few hours to several days.

C. botulinum and some chemicals affect the nervous system, causing symptoms such as

- headache

- tingling or numbness of the skin

- blurred vision

- weakness

- dizziness

- paralysis

What Are The Complications Of Foodborne Illnesses?

Foodborne illnesses may lead to dehydration, hemolytic uremic syndrome (HUS), and other complications. Acute foodborne illnesses may also lead to chronic—or long lasting—health problems.

Dehydration

When someone does not drink enough fluids to replace those that are lost through vomiting and diarrhea, dehydration can result. When dehydrated, the body lacks enough fluid and electrolytes—minerals in salts, including sodium, potassium, and chloride—to function properly. Infants, children, older adults, and people with weak immune systems have the greatest risk of becoming dehydrated.

Signs of dehydration are

- excessive thirst

- infrequent urination

- dark-colored urine

- lethargy, dizziness, or faintness

Signs of dehydration in infants and young children are

- dry mouth and tongue

- lack of tears when crying

- no wet diapers for 3 hours or more

- high fever

- unusually cranky or drowsy behavior

- sunken eyes, cheeks, or soft spot in the skull

Also, when people are dehydrated, their skin does not flatten back to normal right away after being gently pinched and released.

> Severe dehydration may require intravenous fluids and hospitalization. Untreated severe dehydration can cause serious health problems such as organ damage, shock, or coma—a sleeplike state in which a person is not conscious.

Hemolytic Uremic Syndrome (HUS)

Hemolytic uremic syndrome is a rare disease that mostly affects children younger than 10 years of age. HUS develops when *E. coli* bacteria lodged in the digestive tract make toxins that enter the bloodstream. The toxins start to destroy red blood cells, which help the blood to clot, and the lining of the blood vessels.

In the United States, *E. coli O157:H7* infection is the most common cause of HUS, but infection with other strains of *E. coli*, other bacteria, and viruses may also cause HUS. A recent study found that about 6 percent of people with *E. coli O157:H7* infections developed HUS. Children younger than age 5 have the highest risk, but females and people age 60 and older also have increased risk.

Symptoms of *E. coli O157:H7* infection include diarrhea, which may be bloody, and abdominal pain, often accompanied by nausea, vomiting, and fever. Up to a week after *E. coli* symptoms appear, symptoms of HUS may develop, including irritability, paleness, and decreased urination. HUS may lead to acute renal failure, which is a sudden and temporary loss of kidney function. HUS may also affect other organs and the central nervous system. Most people who develop HUS recover with treatment. Research shows that in the United States between 2000 and 2006, fewer than 5 percent of people who developed HUS died of the disorder. Older adults had the highest mortality rate—about one-third of people age 60 and older who developed HUS died.

Studies have shown that some children who recover from HUS develop chronic complications, including kidney problems, high blood pressure, and diabetes.

Other Complications

Some foodborne illnesses lead to other serious complications. For example, *C. botulinum* and certain chemicals in fish and seafood can paralyze the muscles that control breathing. *L. monocytogenes* can cause spontaneous abortion or stillbirth in pregnant women.

Research suggests that acute foodborne illnesses may lead to chronic disorders, including

- **reactive arthritis,** a type of joint inflammation that usually affects the knees, ankles, or feet. Some people develop this disorder following foodborne illnesses caused by certain bacteria, including *C. jejuni* and *Salmonella*. Reactive arthritis usually lasts fewer than 6 months, but this condition may recur or become chronic arthritis.

- **irritable bowel syndrome (IBS),** a disorder of unknown cause that is associated with abdominal pain, bloating, and diarrhea or constipation or both. Foodborne illnesses caused by bacteria increase the risk of developing IBS.

- **Guillain-Barré syndrome,** a disorder characterized by muscle weakness or paralysis that begins in the lower body and progresses to the upper body. This syndrome may occur after foodborne illnesses caused by bacteria, most commonly *C. jejuni*. Most people recover in 6 to 12 months.

A recent study found that adults who had recovered from *E. coli O157:H7* infections had increased risks of high blood pressure, kidney problems, and cardiovascular disease.

When Should People With Foodborne Illnesses See A Healthcare Provider?

People with any of the following symptoms should see a healthcare provider immediately:

- Signs of dehydration
- Prolonged vomiting that prevents keeping liquids down
- Diarrhea for more than 2 days in adults or for more than 24 hours in children
- Severe pain in the abdomen or rectum
- A fever higher than 101 degrees
- Stools containing blood or pus
- Stools that are black and tarry
- Nervous system symptoms
- Signs of HUS

If a child has a foodborne illness, parents or guardians should not hesitate to call a healthcare provider for advice.

How Are Foodborne Illnesses Diagnosed?

To diagnose foodborne illnesses, healthcare providers ask about symptoms, foods and beverages recently consumed, and medical history. Healthcare providers will also perform a physical examination to look for signs of illness.

Diagnostic tests for foodborne illnesses may include a stool culture, in which a sample of stool is analyzed in a laboratory to check for signs of infections or diseases. A sample of vomit or a sample of the suspected food, if available, may also be tested. A healthcare provider may perform additional medical tests to rule out diseases and disorders that cause symptoms similar to the symptoms of foodborne illnesses.

If symptoms of foodborne illnesses are mild and last only a short time, diagnostic tests are usually not necessary.

How Are Foodborne Illnesses Treated?

The only treatment needed for most foodborne illnesses is replacing lost fluids and electrolytes to prevent dehydration.

Over-the-counter medications such as loperamide (Imodium) and bismuth subsalicylate (Pepto-Bismol and Kaopectate) may help stop diarrhea in adults. However, people with bloody diarrhea—a sign of bacterial or parasitic infection—should not use these medications. If diarrhea is caused by bacteria or parasites, over-the-counter medications may prolong the problem. Medications to treat diarrhea in adults can be dangerous for infants and children and should only be given with a healthcare provider's guidance.

If the specific cause of the foodborne illness is diagnosed, a healthcare provider may prescribe medications, such as antibiotics, to treat the illness.

Hospitalization may be required to treat lifethreatening symptoms and complications, such as paralysis, severe dehydration, and HUS.

Eating, Diet, And Nutrition

The following steps may help relieve the symptoms of foodborne illnesses and prevent dehydration in adults:

- drinking plenty of liquids such as fruit juices, sports drinks, caffeine-free soft drinks, and broths to replace fluids and electrolytes

- sipping small amounts of clear liquids or sucking on ice chips if vomiting is still a problem

- gradually reintroducing food, starting with bland, easy-to-digest foods such as rice, potatoes, toast or bread, cereal, lean meat, applesauce, and bananas

- avoiding fatty foods, sugary foods, dairy products, caffeine, and alcohol until recovery is complete

Infants and children present special concerns. Infants and children are likely to become dehydrated more quickly from diarrhea and vomiting because of their smaller body size. The following steps may help relieve symptoms and prevent dehydration in infants and children:

- giving oral rehydration solutions such as Pedialyte, Naturalyte, Infalyte, and CeraLyte to prevent dehydration

- giving food as soon as the child is hungry

- giving infants breast milk or fullstrength formula, as usual, along with oral rehydration solutions

Older adults and adults with weak immune systems should also drink oral rehydration solutions to prevent dehydration.

How Are Foodborne Illnesses Prevented?

Foodborne illnesses can be prevented by properly storing, cooking, cleaning, and handling foods.

- Raw and cooked perishable foods—foods that can spoil—should be refrigerated or frozen promptly. If perishable foods stand at room temperature for more than 2 hours, they may not be safe to eat. Refrigerators should be set at 40 degrees or lower and freezers should be set at 0 degrees.

- Foods should be cooked long enough and at a high enough temperature to kill the harmful bacteria that cause illnesses. A meat thermometer should be used to ensure foods are cooked to the appropriate internal temperature:

  - 145 degrees for roasts, steaks, and chops of beef, veal, pork, and lamb, followed by 3 minutes of rest time after the meat is removed from the heat source

  - 160 degrees for ground beef, veal, pork, and lamb

  - 165 degrees for poultry

- Cold foods should be kept cold and hot foods should be kept hot.

- Fruits and vegetables should be washed under running water just before eating, cutting, or cooking. A produce brush can be used under running water to clean fruits and vegetables with firm skin.

- Raw meat, poultry, seafood, and their juices should be kept away from other foods.

- People should wash their hands for at least 20 seconds with warm, soapy water before and after handling raw meat, poultry, fish, shellfish, produce, or eggs. People should also wash their hands after using the bathroom, changing diapers, or touching animals.

- Utensils and surfaces should be washed with hot, soapy water before and after they are used to prepare food. Diluted bleach—1 teaspoon of bleach to 1 quart of hot water—can also be used to sanitize utensils and surfaces.

Chapter 58

Understanding Eating Disorders

Eating disorders are so common in America that 1 or 2 out of every 100 students will struggle with one. Each year, thousands of teens develop eating disorders, or problems with weight, eating, or body image.

Eating disorders are more than just going on a diet to lose weight or trying to exercise every day. They represent extremes in eating behavior and ways of thinking about eating—the diet that never ends and gradually gets more restrictive, for example. Or the person who can't go out with friends because he or she thinks it's more important to go running to work off a snack eaten earlier.

The most common eating disorders are anorexia nervosa and bulimia nervosa (usually called simply "anorexia" and "bulimia"). But other food-related disorders, like avoidant/restrictive food intake disorder, binge eating, body image disorders, and food phobias, are becoming more and more commonly identified.

Anorexia

People with anorexia have a real fear of weight gain and a distorted view of their body size and shape. As a result, they eat very little and can become dangerously underweight. Many teens with anorexia restrict their food intake by dieting, fasting, or excessive exercise. They hardly eat at all—and the small amount of food they do eat becomes an obsession in terms of calorie counting or trying to eat as little as possible.

About This Chapter: Information in this chapter is excerpted from "Eating Disorders," © 1995–2016. The Nemours Foundation/KidsHealth®. Reprinted with permission.

Others with anorexia may start binge eating and purging—eating a lot of food and then trying to get rid of the calories by making themselves throw up, using some type of medication or laxatives, or exercising excessively, or some combination of these.

Bulimia

Bulimia is similar to anorexia. With bulimia, people might binge eat (eat to excess) and then try to compensate in extreme ways, such as making themselves throw up or exercising all the time, to prevent weight gain. Over time, these steps can be dangerous—both physically and emotionally. They can also lead to compulsive behaviors (ones that are hard to stop).

To have bulimia, a person must be binging and purging regularly, at least once a week for a couple of months. Binge eating is different from going to a party and "pigging out" on pizza, then deciding to go to the gym the next day and eat more healthfully

People with bulimia eat a large amount of food (often junk food) at once, usually in secret. Sometimes they eat food that is not cooked or might be still frozen, or retrieve food from the trash. They typically feel powerless to stop the eating and can only stop once they're too full to eat any more, or they may have to go to extreme measures (like pouring salt all over a dessert to make it inedible) in order to get themselves to stop eating. Most people with bulimia then purge by vomiting, but also may use laxatives or excessive exercise.

Although anorexia and bulimia are very similar, people with anorexia are usually very thin and underweight, but those with bulimia may be an average weight or can be overweight.

Binge Eating Disorder

Binge eating disorder is similar to anorexia and bulimia because a person binges regularly on food (at least once a week, but typically more often). But, unlike the other eating disorders, a person with binge eating disorder does not try to "compensate" by purging the food.

Anorexia, bulimia, and binge eating disorder all involve unhealthy eating patterns that begin gradually and build to the point where a person feels unable to control them.

Avoidant/Restrictive Food Intake Disorder (ARFID)

ARFID is a new term that some people think just means "picky eating," but a number of other eating issues can also cause it. People with ARFID don't have anorexia or bulimia, but they still struggle with eating and as a result don't eat enough to keep a healthy body weight.

Types of eating problems that might be considered ARFID include:

- difficulty digesting certain foods

- avoiding certain colors or textures of food

- eating only very small portions

- having no appetite

- being afraid to eat after a frightening episode of choking or vomiting

Because they don't get enough nutrition in their diet, people with ARFID lose weight, or, if they're younger kids, they may not gain weight or grow as expected. Many people with ARFID need supplements each day to get the right amount of nutrition and calories.

People with ARFID also might have issues in their day-to-day lives, at school, or with their friends because of their eating problems. For example, they might avoid going out to eat or eating lunch at school, or it might take so long to eat that they're late for school or don't have time to do their homework.

Some people with ARFID may go on to develop another eating disorder, such as anorexia or bulimia.

Signs Of Anorexia And Bulimia

Sometimes a person with anorexia or bulimia starts out just trying to lose some weight or hoping to get in shape. But the urge to eat less or to purge or over-exercise gets "addictive" and becomes too hard to stop.

Not Just a Girl Thing

More guys are seeking help for eating disorders. Guys with eating disorders tend to focus more on athletic appearance or success than on just looking thin.

Teens with anorexia or bulimia often feel intense fear of being fat or think that they're fat when they are not. Those with anorexia may weigh food before eating it or compulsively count the calories of everything. People to whom this seems "normal" or "cool" or who wish that others would leave them alone so they can just diet and be thin might have a serious problem.

How do you know for sure that someone is struggling with anorexia or bulimia? You can't tell just by looking—a person who loses a lot of weight might have another health condition or could be losing weight through healthy eating and exercise.

But there are some signs to watch for that might indicate a person has anorexia or bulimia.

Someone With Anorexia Might:

- become very thin, frail, or emaciated

- be obsessed with eating, food, and weight control

- weigh herself or himself repeatedly

- deliberately "water load" when going to see a health professional to get weighed

- count or portion food carefully

- only eat certain foods, avoiding foods like dairy, meat, wheat, etc. (of course, lots of people who are allergic to a particular food or are vegetarians avoid certain foods)

- exercise excessively

- feel fat

- withdraw from social activities, especially meals and celebrations involving food

- be depressed, lethargic (lacking in energy), and feel cold a lot

Someone With Bulimia Might:

- fear weight gain

- be intensely unhappy with body size, shape, and weight

- make excuses to go to the bathroom immediately after meals

- only eat diet or low-fat foods (except during binges)

- regularly buy laxatives, diuretics, or enemas

- spend most of his or her time working out or trying to work off calories

- withdraw from social activities, especially meals and celebrations involving food

What Causes Eating Disorders?

No one is really sure what causes eating disorders, although there are many theories about it. Many people who develop an eating disorder are between 13 and 17 years old. This is a time of emotional and physical changes, academic pressures, and a greater degree of peer pressure.

Although there is a sense of greater independence during the teen years, teens might feel that they are not in control of their personal freedom and, sometimes, of their bodies. This can be especially true during puberty.

For girls, even though it's completely normal (and necessary) to gain some additional body fat during puberty, some respond to this change by becoming very fearful of their new weight. They might mistakenly feel compelled to get rid of it any way they can.

A Not-So-Perfect Picture

We're overloaded by images of thin celebrities—people who often weigh far less than their healthy weight (and who may have histories of eating disorders). So it's easy to see why people may develop a fear of weight gain, even if that gain is temporary and healthy.

When you combine the pressure to be like celebrity role models with the fact that bodies grow and change during puberty, it's not hard to see why some teens develop a negative view of themselves. Celebrity teens and athletes conform to the "Hollywood ideal"—girls are petite and skinny, and guys are athletic and muscular, and these body types are popular not only in Hollywood but also in high school.

Many people with eating disorders also can be depressed or anxious, or have other mental health problems such as obsessive compulsive disorder (OCD). There is also evidence that eating disorders may run in families. Although part of this may be genetics, it's also because we learn our values and behaviors from our families.

Sports And Eating Disorders

Athletes and dancers are particularly vulnerable to developing eating disorders around the time of puberty, as they may want to stop or suppress growth (both height and weight).

Coaches, family members, and others may encourage teens in certain sports—such as gymnastics, ice skating, and ballet—to be as thin as possible. Some athletes and runners are also encouraged to weigh less or shed body fat at a time when they are biologically destined to gain it.

Effects Of Eating Disorders

Eating disorders are serious medical illnesses. They often go along with other problems such as stress, anxiety, depression, and substance use. Eating disorders can lead to the development of serious physical health problems, such as heart conditions or kidney failure.

Someone whose body weight is at least 15 percent less than the average weight for that person's height may not have enough body fat to keep organs and other body parts healthy. In severe cases, eating disorders can lead to severe malnutrition and even death.

With anorexia, the body goes into starvation mode, and the lack of nutrition can affect the body in many ways:

- a drop in blood pressure, pulse, and breathing rate

- hair loss and fingernail breakage

- loss of periods

- lanugo hair—a soft hair that can grow all over the skin

- lightheadedness and inability to concentrate

- anemia

- swollen joints

- brittle bones

With bulimia, constant vomiting and lack of nutrients can cause these problems:

- constant stomach pain

- damage to the stomach and kidneys

- tooth decay (from exposure to stomach acids)

- "chipmunk cheeks," when the salivary glands permanently expand from throwing up so often

- loss of periods

- loss of the mineral potassium (this can contribute to heart problems and even death)

A person with binge eating disorder who gains a lot of weight is at risk of developing diabetes, heart disease, and some of the other diseases associated with being overweight.

The emotional pain of an eating disorder can take its toll, too. When someone becomes obsessed with weight, it's hard to concentrate on much else. It can be exhausting and overwhelming to monitor food intake and exercise, and be in a constant state of stress about food and how your body looks. It's easy to see why when you develop an eating disorder you could become withdrawn and less social. It gets too hard to join in on snacks and meals with friends or families, or too hard to stop the addictive exercising or working out to have fun.

Having an eating disorder also can use up a lot of mental energy planning what to eat, how to avoid food, planning a binge, getting money to buy food or laxatives or other medications, making up reasons to use the bathroom after meals, or figuring out how to tell people around you that you want to be alone after a meal.

Treatment For Eating Disorders

Fortunately, eating disorders can be treated. People with eating disorders can get well and gradually learn to eat well and more like their family and friends again. Eating disorders involve both the mind and body. So medical doctors, mental health professionals, and dietitians will often be involved in a person's treatment and recovery.

Therapy or counseling is a very important part of getting better—in many cases, family therapy is one of the keys to eating healthily again. Parents and other family members are important in supporting people who have to regain weight that they are afraid of, or to learn to accept the body shape that their culture, genes, and lifestyle allows for.

If you want to talk to someone about eating disorders but are unable or not ready to talk to a parent or close family member, try reaching out to a friend, teacher, school nurse or counselor, coach, neighbor, your doctor, or another trusted adult.

Learning to be comfortable at your healthy weight is a process. It takes time to unlearn some behaviors and relearn others. Be patient, you can learn to like your body, understand your eating behaviors, and figure out the relationship between feelings and eating—all the tools you need to feel in control and to like and accept yourself for who you are.

Don't Wait to Get Help

Like all bad habits, unhealthy eating patterns become harder to break the longer a person does them. The most critical thing about treating eating disorders is to recognize and address the problem as soon as possible.

Eating disorders can do a lot of damage to the body and mind if left untreated, and they don't get better by themselves.

Part Seven
If You Need More Information

Chapter 59
Cooking Tips And Resources

Healthy Cooking And Snacking

Food doesn't have to be high in fat to be good. Get the **whole family** to help slice, dice, and chop, and learn how to cut fat and calories in some foods. You'd be surprised how easy heart healthy cooking and snacking can be.

In this chapter you'll find ideas for healthy snacks, tips for healthy cooking, and food options with less fat and fewer calories.

Healthy Family Snacks

Try these tips for quick and easy snacks:

- Toss sliced apples, berries, bananas, or whole-grain cereal on top of fat-free or low-fat yogurt.

- Put a slice of fat-free or low-fat cheese on top of whole-grain crackers.

- Make a whole-wheat pita pocket with hummus, lettuce, tomato, and cucumber.

- Pop some fat-free or low-fat popcorn.

- Microwave or toast a soft whole grain tortilla with fat-free or low-fat cheese and sliced peppers and mushrooms to make a mini-burrito or quesadilla.

- Drink fat-free or low-fat chocolate milk (blend it with a banana or strawberries and some ice for a smoothie).

About This Chapter: Information in this chapter is excerpted from "Healthy Cooking and Snacking," National Heart, Lung, and Blood Institute (NHLBI), February 13, 2013.

Healthy Cooking Tips

Make a few changes in the kitchen and you'll be eating healthy in no time.

Tips For Reducing Fat

- Instead of frying, try baking, broiling, boiling, or microwaving.

- Choose fat-free or low-fat milk products, salad dressings, and mayonnaise.

- Add salsa on a baked potato instead of butter or sour cream.

- Remove skin from poultry (like chicken or turkey) and do not eat it.

- Cool soups and gravies and skim off fat before reheating them.

Tips For Reducing Sugar

- Serve fruit instead of cookies or ice cream for dessert.

- Eat fruits canned in their own juice rather than syrup.

- Reduce sugar in recipes by 1/4 to 1/3. If a recipe says 1 cup, use 2/3 cup.

- To enhance the flavor when sugar is reduced, add vanilla, cinnamon, or nutmeg.

Healthy Baking And Cooking Substitutes

Cut the fat and sugar in your meals by using these substitutes.

Table 59.1. Cooking Substitutes

Instead of:	Substitute:
1 cup cream	1 cup evaporated fat-free milk
1 cup butter, margarine, or oil	1/2 cup apple butter or applesauce
1 egg	2 egg whites or 1/4 cup egg substitute
Pastry dough	Graham cracker crumb crust
Butter, margarine, or vegetable oil for sautéing	Cooking spray, chicken broth, or a small amount of olive oil
Bacon	Lean turkey bacon
Ground beef	Extra lean ground beef or ground turkey breast
Sour cream	Fat-free sour cream
1 cup chocolate chips	1/4 - 1/2 cup mini chocolate chips

Table 59.1. Continued

Instead of:	Substitute:
1 cup sugar	3/4 cup sugar (this works with nearly everything except yeast breads)
1 cup mayonnaise	1 cup fat-free or reduced-fat mayonnaise
1 cup whole milk	1 cup fat-free milk
1 cup cream cheese	1/2 cup ricotta cheese pureed with 1/2 cup fat-free cream cheese
Oil and vinegar dressing with 3 parts oil to 1 part vinegar	1 part olive oil + 1 part vinegar (preferably a flavored vinegar, such as balsamic) + 1 part orange juice
Unsweetened baking chocolate (1 ounce)	3 tablespoons unsweetened cocoa powder + 1 tablespoon vegetable oil or margarine

Note: Substitute the ingredients in your own favorite recipes to lower the amounts of fat, added sugar, and calories.

Chapter 60

Eat Smart And Be Active As You Grow—Tips For Teen Guys

Feed your growing body by making better food choices today as a teen and as you continue to grow into your twenties. Make time to be physically active every day to help you be fit and healthy as you grow.

1. **Get over the idea of magic foods**

   There are no magic foods to eat for good health. Teen guys need to eat foods such as vegetables, fruits, whole grains, protein foods, and fat-free or low-fat dairy foods. Choose protein foods like unsalted nuts, beans, lean meats, and fish. SuperTracker (www.choosemyplate.gov/MyPlate) will show if you are getting the nutrients you need for growth.

2. **Always hungry?**

   Whole grains that provide fiber can give you a feeling of fullness and provide key nutrients. Choose half your grains as whole grains. Eat whole-wheat breads, pasta, and brown rice instead of white bread, rice, or other refined grains. Also, choose vegetables and fruits when you need to "fill-up."

3. **Keep water handy**

   Water is a better option than many other drink choices. Keep a water bottle in your backpack and at your desk to satisfy your thirst. Skip soda, fruit drinks, and energy and sports drinks. They are sugar-sweetened and have few nutrients.

About This Chapter: Information in this chapter is excerpted from "Choose the Foods You Need to Grow," ChooseMyPlate.gov, U.S. Department of Agriculture (USDA), July 11, 2016.

4. **Make a list of favorite foods**

Like green apples more than red apples? Ask your family food shopper to buy quick-to-eat foods for the fridge like mini-carrots, apples, oranges, low-fat cheese slices, or yogurt. And also try dried fruit; unsalted nuts; whole-grain breads, cereal, and crackers; and popcorn.

5. **Start cooking often**

Get over being hungry by fixing your own snacks and meals. Learn to make vegetable omelets, bean quesadillas, or a batch of spaghetti. Prepare your own food so you can make healthier meals and snacks. Microwaving frozen pizzas doesn't count as home cooking.

6. **Skip foods that can add unwanted pounds**

Cut back on calories by limiting fatty meats like ribs, bacon, and hot dogs. Some foods are just occasional treats like pizza, cakes, cookies, candies, and ice cream. Check out the calorie content of sugary drinks by reading the Nutrition Facts label. Many 12-ounce sodas contain 10 teaspoons of sugar.

7. **Learn how much food you need**

Teen guys may need more food than most adults, teen girls, and little kids. Go to Super-Tracker.usda.gov. It shows how much food you need based on your age, height, weight, and activity level. It also tracks progress towards fitness goals.

8. **Check Nutrition Facts labels**

To grow, your body needs vitamins and minerals. Calcium and vitamin D are especially important for your growing bones. Read Nutrition Facts labels for calcium. Dairy foods provide the minerals your bones need to grow.

9. **Strengthen your muscles**

Work on strengthening and aerobic activities. Work out at least 10 minutes at a time to see a better you. However, you need to get at least 60 minutes of physical activity every day.

10. **Fill your plate like MyPlate**

MyPlate (www.choosemyplate.gov/MyPlate) is based on the *Dietary Guidelines for Americans*.

Chapter 61

Eat Smart And Be Active As You Grow—Tips For Teen Girls

Young girls, ages 10 to 19, have a lot of changes going on in their bodies. Building healthier habits will help you—now as a growing teen—and later in life. Growing up means you are in charge of foods you eat and the time you spend being physically active every day.

1. **Build strong bones**

   A good diet and regular physical activity can build strong bones throughout your life. Choose fat-free or low-fat milk, cheeses, and yogurt to get the vitamin D and calcium your growing bones need. Strengthen your bones three times a week doing activities such as running, gymnastics, and skating.

2. **Cut back on sweets**

   Cut back on sugary drinks. Many 12-ounce cans of soda have 10 teaspoons of sugar in them. Drink water when you are thirsty. Sipping water and cutting back on cakes, candies, and sweets helps to maintain a healthy weight.

3. **Power up with whole grain**

   Fuel your body with nutrient-packed whole-grain foods. Make sure that at least half your grain foods are whole grains such as brown rice, whole-wheat breads, and popcorn.

4. **Choose vegetables rich in color**

   Brighten your plate with vegetables that are red, orange, or dark green. Try acorn squash, cherry tomatoes, or sweet potatoes. Spinach and beans also provide vitamins like folate and minerals like potassium that are essential for healthy growth.

About This Chapter: Information in this chapter is excerpted from "Eat Smart and Be Active as You Grow," ChooseMyPlate.gov, U.S. Department of Agriculture (USDA), July 11, 2016.

5. **Check Nutrition Facts labels for iron**

   Read Nutrition Facts labels to find foods containing iron. Most protein foods like meat, poultry, eggs, and beans have iron, and so do fortified breakfast cereals and breads.

6. **Be a healthy role model**

   Encourage your friends to practice healthier habits. Share what you do to work through challenges. Keep your computer and TV time to less than 2 hours a day (unless it's school work).

7. **Try something new**

   Keep healthy eating fun by picking out new foods you've never tried before like lentils, mango, quinoa, or kale.

8. **Make moving part of every event**

   Being active makes everyone feel good. Aim for 60 minutes of physical activity each day. Move your body often. Dancing, playing active games, walking to school with friends, swimming, and biking are only a few fun ways to be active. Also, try activities that target the muscles in your arms and legs.

9. **Include all food groups daily**

   Use MyPlate (www.choosemyplate.gov/MyPlate) as your guide to include all food groups each day.

10. **Everyone has different needs**

    Get nutrition information based on your age, gender, height, weight, and physical activity level. Use SuperTracker (www.supertracker.usda.gov) to find your calorie level, choose the foods you need, and track progress toward your goals.

Chapter 62
Resources For Dietary Information

Academy of Nutrition and Dietetics (AND)
120 S. Riverside Plaza, Ste. 2000
Chicago, IL 60606-6995
Toll-Free: 800-877-1600
Phone: 312-899-0040
Fax: 312-899-4873
Website: www.eatright.org
E-mail: webstrategy@eatright.org

American Diabetes Association (ADA)
1701 N. Beauregard St.
Alexandria, VA 22311
Toll-Free: 800-DIABETES (800-342-2383)
Website: www.diabetes.com

Asthma and Allergy Foundation of America (AAFA)
8201 Corporate Dr., Ste. 1000
Landover, MD 20785
Toll-Free: 800-7-ASTHMA
(800-727-8462)
Website: www.aafa.org
E-mail: info@aafa.org

Celiac Disease Foundation (CDF)
20350 Ventura Blvd., Ste. 240
Woodland Hills, CA 91364
Phone: 818-716-1513
Fax: 818-267-5577
Website: www.celiac.org
E-mail: cdf@celiac.org

Center for Nutrition Policy and Promotion (CNPP)
3101 Park Center Dr.
Alexandria, VA 22302-1594
Website: www.choosemyplate.gov
E-mail: support@cnpp.usda.gov

Center for Science in the Public Interest (CSPI)
1220 L St. N.W.
Ste. 300
Washington, DC 20009
Phone: 202-332-9110
Fax: 202-265-4954
Website: www.cspinet.org
E-mail: cspi@cspinet.org

About This Chapter: Information in this chapter was compiled from many sources deemed reliable; inclusion does not constitute endorsement. All contact information was verified and updated in September 2016.

Eating Disorder Referral and Information Center

2923 Sandy Pt.
Ste. 6
Del Mar, CA 92014-2052
Phone: 858-792-7463
Fax: 858-220-7417
Website: www.edreferral.com
E-mail: edreferral@aol.com

Eunice Kennedy Shriver National Institute of Child Health and Human Development (NICHD)

31 Center Dr.
Rm. 2A32
Bethesda, MD 20892-2425
Toll-Free: 800-370-2943
Phone: 301-496-5133
Fax: 301-496-7101
Website: www.nichd.nih.gov
E-mail:
NICHDInformationResourceCenter@mail.nih.gov

Food Allergy and Research Education, Inc. (FARE)

7925 Jones Branch Dr.
Ste. 1100
McLean, VA 22102
Toll-Free: 800-929-4040
Fax: 703-691-2713
Website: www.foodallergy.org
E-mail: info@foodallergy.org

Food and Nutrition Information Center (FNIC)

USDA Agriculture Research Service
10301 Baltimore Ave.
Rm. 108
Beltsville, MD 20705
Phone: 301-504-5414
Fax: 301-504-6409
Website: fnic.nal.usda.gov
E-mail: FNIC@ars.usda.gov

Food Safety and Inspection Service (FSIS)

United States Department of Agriculture
1400 Independence Ave. S.W.
Washington, DC 20250-3700
Phone: 202-720-9113
Website: www.fsis.usda.gov
E-mail: fsis.webmaster@usda.gov

Institute of Food Technologists

525 W. Van Buren, Ste. 1000
Chicago, IL 60607
Toll-Free: 800-IFT-FOOD (800-438-3663)
Phone: 312-782-8424
Fax: 312-782-8348
Website: www.ift.org
Email: info@ift.org

International Food Information Council (IFIC) Foundation

1100 Connecticut Ave. N.W., Ste. 430
Washington, DC 20036
Phone: 202-296-6540
Website: www.foodinsight.org
E-mail: info@foodinsight.org

National Association of Anorexia Nervosa and Associated Disorders (ANAD)

750 E. Diehl Rd., Ste. 127
Naperville, IL 60563
Phone: 630-577-1333
Fax: 630-577-1323
Website: www.anad.org
E-mail: anadhelp@anad.org

National Center for Complementary and Alternative Medicine (NCCAM)

NCCAM Clearinghouse
P.O. Box 7923
Gaithersburg, MD 20898-7923
Toll-Free: 888-644-6226
TTY: 866-464-3615
Fax: 866-464-3616
Website: nccih.nih.gov
E-mail: info@nccam.nih.gov

National Diabetes Education Program (NDEP)

1 Diabetes Way
Bethesda, MD 20814-9692
Toll-Free: 888-693-6337
Phone: 301-496-3583
Website: www.ndep.nih.gov
E-mail:ndep@mail.nih.gov

National Eating Disorders Association (NEDA)

603 Stewart St., Ste. 803
Seattle, WA 98101
Toll-Free: 800-931-2237
Phone: 206-382-3587
Fax: 206-829-8501
Website: www.nationaleatingdisorders.org
E-mail: info@myneda.org

National Heart, Lung, and Blood Institute (NHLBI)

NHLBI Health Information Center
P.O. Box 30105
Bethesda, MD 20824-0105
Phone: 301-592-8573
TTY: 240-629-3255
Website: www.nhlbi.nih.gov
E-mail: NHLBIinfo@nhlbi.nih.gov

Obesity Society

8757 Georgia Ave., Ste. 1320
Silver Spring, MD 20910
Toll Free: 800-974-3084
Phone: 301-563-6526
Fax: 301-563-6595
Website: www.obesity.org

Office of Dietary Supplements

National Institutes of Health
6100 Executive Blvd.
Rm. 3B01, MSC 7517
Bethesda, MD 20892-7517
Phone: 301-435-2920
Fax: 301-480-1845
Website: ods.od.nih.gov
E-mail: ods@nih.gov

U.S. Department of Agriculture

1400 Independence Ave. S.W.
Washington, DC 20250
Phone: 202-720-2791
Website: www.usda.gov

U.S. Food and Drug Administration (FDA)

Consumer Inquiries
10903 New Hampshire Ave.
Silver Spring, MD 20993
Toll-Free: 888-INFO-FDA (888-463-6332)
Website: www.fda.gov
E-mail: ConsumerInfo@fda.hhs.gov

The Vegetarian Resource Group (VRG)
P.O. Box 1463
Baltimore, MD 21203
Phone: 410-366-8343
Website: www.vrg.org
E-mail: vrg@vrg.org

Weight-Control Information Network (WIN)
1 WIN Way
Bethesda, MD 20892-3665
Toll-Free: 877-946-4627
Fax: 202-828-1028
Website: win.niddk.nih.gov
E-mail: win@info.niddk.nih.gov

Interactive Tools and Other Online Resources

Ask the Dietitian® Calculators
Healthy Eating for Life Plan®
Website: www.dietitian.com/calcbody.php

Body and Mind: Food and Nutrition
Centers for Disease Control and Prevention
Website: www.cdc.gov/bam/nutrition

Body Mass Index Calculator
National Heart, Lung, and Blood Institute
Website: www.nhlbi.nih.gov/health/educational/lose_wt/BMI/bmicalc.htm

Calcium Quiz—What's Your Calcium Intake?
Dairy Council of California
Website: www.dairycouncilofca.org/Tools/CalciumQuiz

Eat Local: Search for Local Produce or Farmers Markets
National Resources Defense Council
Website: www.simplesteps.org/eat-local

Get Moving! Calculate the Number of Calories Burned
Calorie Control Council
Website: www.caloriecontrol.org/exercalc.html

Girl's Health: Nutrition
Office on Women's Health
Website: www.girlshealth.gov/nutrition

Farmers Market Search
USDA, Agricultural Marketing Service
Website: apps.ams.usda.gov/FarmersMarkets

Fruits and Veggies Matter Interactive Tools
Centers for Disease Control and Prevention
Website: www.fruitsandveggies matter.gov/activities/index.html

Healthy Dining Finder
Website: www.healthydiningfinder.com

Kidnetic
International Food Information Council
Website: kidnetic.com

MyPlate
U.S. Department of Agriculture
Website: www.choosemyplate.gov

Nutrition Explorations
Website: www.nutritionexplorations.org

Nutrition.gov
National Agricultural Library
Website: www.nutrition.gov

Personal Nutrition Planner from Meals Matter
Dairy Council of California
Website: www.mealsmatter.org

Rate Your Restaurant Diet
Center for Science in the Public Interest
Website: www.cspinet.org/nah/quiz/index.html

Spark Teens
Website: www.sparkteens.com

Chapter 63
Resources For Fitness Information

Action for Healthy Kids (AFHK)
4711 W. Golf Rd.
Ste. 625
Skokie, IL 60076
Toll-Free: 800-416-5136
Website: www.actionforhealthykids.org
E-mail: info@actionforhealthykids.org

Aerobics and Fitness Association of America (AFAA)
1750 E. Northrop Blvd.
Ste. 200
Chandler, AZ 85286-1744
Toll-Free: 800-446-2322
Website: www.afaa.com
E-mail: customerservice@afaa.com

American Academy of Orthopaedic Surgeons (AAOS)
9400 W. Higgins Rd.
Rosemont, IL 60018-4262
Phone: 847-823-7186
Fax: 847-823-8125
Website: www.aaos.org
E-mail:customerservice@aaos.org

American College of Sports Medicine (ACSM)
401 W. Michigan St.
P.O. Box 1440
Indianapolis, IN 46206-1440
Phone: 317-637-9200
Fax: 317-634-7817
Website: www.acsm.org

American Council on Exercise (ACE)
4851 Paramount Dr.
San Diego, CA 92123
Toll-Free: 888-825-3636
Phone: 858-576-6500
Fax: 858-576-6564
Website: www.acefitness.org
E-mail: support@acefitness.org

American Health and Fitness Alliance
P.O. Box 20750
New York, NY 10021
Phone: 212-573-9200
Fax: 212-808-0765
Website: www.bbb.org

About This Chapter: Information in this chapter was compiled from many sources deemed reliable; inclusion does not constitute endorsement. All contact information was verified and updated in September 2016.

American Heart Association (AHA)
7272 Greenville Ave.
Dallas, TX 75231
Toll-Free: 800-242-8721
Website: www.americanheart.org

American Orthopaedic Society for Sports Medicine (AOSSM)
9400 W. Higgins Rd.
Ste. 300
Rosemont, IL 60018
Toll-Free: 877-321-3500
Phone: 847-292-4900
Fax: 847-292-4905
Website: www.sportsmed.org
E-mail: aossm@aossm.org

American Physical Therapy Association (APTA)
1111 N. Fairfax St.
Alexandria, VA 22314-1488
Toll-Free: 800-999-2782
Phone: 703-684-2782
TDD: 703-683-6748
Fax: 703-684-7343
Website: www.apta.org
E-mail: webmaSte.r@apta.org

American Physiological Society (APS)
9650 Rockville Pike
Bethesda, MD 20814-3991
Phone: 301-634-7164
Fax: 301-634-7241
Website: www.the-aps.org

American Running Association (ARA)
4405 E.W. Hwy.
Ste. 405
Bethesda, MD 20814
Phone: 800-776-2732 ext. 13 or ext. 12
Fax: 301-913-9520
Website: www.americanrunning.org

American Society of Exercise Physiologists (ASEP)
The College of St. Scholastica
1200 Kenwood Ave.
Duluth, MN 55811
Phone: 218-723-6297
Fax: 218-723-6472
Website: www.asep.org

Aquatic Exercise Association (AEA)
P.O. Box 1609
Nokomis, FL 34274-1609
Website: www.aeawave.com

Centers for Disease Control and Prevention (CDC)
Division of Nutrition, Physical Activity, and Obesity (DNPAO)
1600 Clifton Rd.
Atlanta, GA 30329-4027
Toll-Free: 800-232-4636
Toll-Free TTY: 888-232-6348
Website: www.cdc.gov
E-mail: cdcinfo@cdc.gov

Disabled Sports USA (DS/USA)
451 Hungerford Dr., Ste. 100
Rockville, MD 20850
Phone: 301-217-0960
Fax: 301-217-0968
Website: www.disabledsportsusa.org
E-mail: info@dsusa.org

Girls Health
200 Independence Ave S.W.
Rm. 712E
Washington, DC 20201
Website: www.girlshealth.gov

IDEA Health & Fitness Association
10190 Telesis Ct.
San Diego, CA 92121
Toll-Free: 800-999-4332, ext. 7
Phone: 858-535-8979, ext. 7
Fax: 619-344-0380
Website: www.ideafit.com
E-mail: contact@ideafit.com

International Fitness Association (IFA)
12472 Lake Underhill Rd., Ste. 341
Orlando, FL 32828
Toll-Free: 800-227-1976
Phone: 407-579-8610
Website: www.fitnessprofessionalonline.com

International Health, Racquet & Sportsclub Association (IHRSA)
70 Fargo St.
Boston, MA 02210
Toll-Free: 800-228-4772
Phone: 617-951-0055
Fax: 617-951-0056
Website: www.ihrsa.org

Kids.gov
Website: www.kids.gov

KidsHealth®
The Nemours Foundation
Website: www.kidshealth.org

National Academy of Sports Medicine (NASM)
1750 E. Northrop Blvd.
Ste. 200
Chandler, AZ 85286-1744
Toll-Free 800-460-6276
International: 1-818-595-1200
Fax: 480-656-3276
Website: www.nasm.org
E-mail: nasmcares@nasm.org

National Alliance for Youth Sports (NAYS)
2050 Vista Pkwy
West Palm Beach, FL 33411
Toll-Free: 800-688-5437
Phone: 561-684-1141
Fax: 561-684-2546
Website: www.nays.org
E-mail: nays@nays.org

National Association for Health and Fitness (NAHF)
65 Niagara Sq.
Rm. 607
Buffalo, NY 14202
Phone: 716-583-0521
Fax: 716-851-4309
Website: healthfinder.gov
E-mail: wellness@city-buffalo.org

National Coalition for Promoting Physical Activity (NCPPA)

1150 Connecticut Ave. N.W.,
Ste. 300
Washington, DC 20036
Website: www.ncppa.org

National Institute for Fitness and Sport (NIFS)

250 University Blvd.
Indianapolis, IN 46202
Phone: 317-274-3432
Fax: 317-274-7408
Website: www.nifs.org

National Institutes of Health (NIH)

9000 Rockville Pike
Bethesda, MD 20892
Phone: 301-496-4000
TTY: 301-402-9612
Website: www.nih.gov
E-mail: NIHinfo@od.nih.gov

National Recreation and Park Association (NRPA)

22377 Belmont Ridge Rd.
Ashburn, VA 20148-4501
Toll-Free: 800-626-6772
Website: www.nrpa.org

National Strength and Conditioning Association (NSCA)

1885 Bob Johnson Dr.
Colorado Springs, CO 80906
Toll-Free: 800-815-6826
Phone: 719-632-6722
Fax: 719-632-6367
Website: www.nsca-lift.org
E-mail: nsca@nsca.com

PE Central

1995 S. Main St.
Ste. 902, P.O. Box 10262
Blacksburg, VA 24060
Phone: 540-953-1043
Fax: 866-776-9170
Website: www.pecentral.org
E-mail: pec@pecentral.org

President's Council on Fitness, Sports, and Nutrition (PCFSN)

1101 Wootton Pkwy
Ste. 560
Rockville, MD 20852
Phone: 240-276-9567
Fax: 240-276-9860
Website: www.fitness.gov
E-mail: fitness@hhs.gov

SmallStep

U.S. Department of Health and Human Services
200 Independence Ave. S.W.
Washington, D.C. 20201
Toll-Free: 877-696-6775
Website: www.hhs.gov

Society of Health and Physical Educators (SHAPE America)

1900 Association Dr.
Reston, VA 20191-1598
Toll-Free: 800-213-7193
Phone: 703-476-3400
Fax: 703 476-9527
Website: www.shapeamerica.org

Womenshealth.gov

200 Independence Ave. S.W.
Washington, DC 20201
Toll-Free: 800-994-9662
Website: www.womenshealth.gov

Women's Sports Foundation (WSF)

Eisenhower Park
1899 Hempstead Tpke
Ste. 400
East Meadow, NY 11554
Toll-Free: 800-227-3988
Phone: 516-542-4700
Fax: 516-542-4716
Website: www.womenssportsfoundation.org
E-mail: Anaylor@
WomensSportsFoundation.org

Index

Index

Page numbers that appear in *Italics* refer to tables or illustrations. Page numbers that have a small 'n' after the page number refer to citation information shown as Notes. Page numbers that appear in **Bold** refer to information contained in boxes within the chapters.

A

"About Child and Teen BMI" (CDC) 229n
Academy of Nutrition and Dietetics (AND), contact 343
acceptable daily intake (ADI), high-intensity sweeteners 154
Ace-K *see* acesulfame potassium
acesulfame potassium (Ace-K)
 high-intensity sweeteners 153
 tabulated *165*
Action for Healthy Kids (AFHK), contact 349
added sugar
 beverage choices 64
 childhood obesity 285
 dairy group 42
 empty calories 59
 fast food 180
 food items to avoid 149
 GO, SLOW, and WHOA foods **207**
 healthy eating pattern 5
 nutrition facts label 21, 187
 overview 151–2
 packaged and restaurant food 282
 protein foods group 48
adequate intakes (AIs)
 chromium 121
 multivitamin/mineral (MVM) supplements 127

ADI *see* acceptable daily intake
advantame, high-intensity sweeteners 153
advertising
 childhood obesity 284
 health fraud 258
Aerobics and Fitness Association of America (AFAA), contact 349
age-related macular degeneration (AMD)
 vitamin A 71
 vitamin C 87
 vitamin E 95
 zinc 117
Agriculture Department *see* U.S. Department of Agriculture
AIs *see* adequate intakes
ALA *see* alpha linolenic acid
"Alcohol and Public Health" (CDC) 209n
alcoholic beverage, alcohol and energy drinks 212
"All about Oils" (USDA) 55n
"All about the Dairy Group" (USDA) 41n
"All about the Fruit Group" (USDA) 35n
"All about the Grains Group" (USDA) 23n
"All about the Protein Foods Group" (USDA) 47n
"All about the Vegetable Group" (USDA) 29n
allergens, preventing food allergy 305
alpha linolenic acid (ALA), omega-3 fatty acids 223
alpha-tocopherol, vitamin E 94

American Academy of Orthopaedic Surgeons (AAOS), contact 349

American College of Sports Medicine (ACSM), contact 349

American Council on Exercise (ACE), contact 349

American Diabetes Association (ADA), contact 343

American Health and Fitness Alliance, contact 349

American Heart Association (AHA), contact 350

American Orthopaedic Society for Sports Medicine (AOSSM), contact 350

American Physical Therapy Association (APTA), contact 350

American Physiological Society (APS), contact 350

American Running Association (ARA), contact 350

American Society of Exercise Physiologists (ASEP), contact 350

anabolic steroids, sports supplements 216

anaphylaxis, exercise-induced food allergy *306*

androstenedione, sports supplements 216

anemia
  anorexia 330
  folate deficiency 75
  grains and nutrients 25
  iron deficiency 109
  vitamin B12 82

anorexia, eating disorders 325

anti-caking agents, tabulated *168*

antidepressant medications, folate effects 76

antioxidants
  food and color ingredients 162
  tabulated *165*
  veganism 222
  vitamin A effects 71
  vitamin C effects 86
  vitamin E effects 95

Aquatic Exercise Association (AEA), contact 350

ARFID *see* avoidant/restrictive food intake disorder

ascorbic acid *see* vitamin C

Ask the Dietitian® Calculators, website address 346

aspartame
  high-intensity sweeteners 153
  tabulated *165*

Asthma and Allergy Foundation of America (AAFA), contact 343

athletes
  eating disorders 329
  energy drink recommendations *212*
  sports supplements 216
  veganism 222

athletic pressure, tips for athletes 218

avoidant/restrictive food intake disorder (ARFID), eating disorders 326

B

B vitamins *see* vitamin B

bacteria
  food and color ingredients 162
  foodborne illnesses 315
  lactose intolerance 307
  tabulated *165*
  vitamin D 89
  vitamin E 93
  vitamin K 98
  zinc 115

baking soda *see* sodium bicarbonate

beans
  calcium and vitamin D *311*
  dairy group 42
  fast food alternatives 196
  healthy eating pattern 5
  protein foods group 47
  starches 299
  tabulated *185*
  vegetable group 29
  vegetarian eating pattern 224

beta-carotene
  color additives 163
  multivitamin and mineral 130
  tabulated *166*
  vitamin A 69
  vitamin C 87
  zinc 117

beverage
  added sugars 151
  alcohol and energy drinks 212
  caloric balance 8
  childhood obesity 285
  food myths 245
  foodborne illnesses 315
  multivitamin/mineral supplements 130
  tabulated *246*

binge eating disorder, eating disorders 326

birth defects
  effects of folate 75
  multivitamin and mineral (MVM) dietary supplements 129
  vitamin A 72

blood glucose
    diabetes 295
    diabetes food pyramid *298*
    fats and sweets 302
blood tests, celiac disease 291
BMI *see* body mass index
BMI calculator 229
BMI percentile 230
Body and Mind: Food and Nutrition, website
  address 346
body image
    eating disorders 325
    overview 237–40
"Body Image and Self-Esteem" (The Nemours
  Foundation/KidsHealth®) 237n
body mass index (BMI)
    food myths 245
    overview 229–32
    see also BMI percentile
Body Mass Index Calculator, website address 346
bone disorders, vitamin D 91
bone health
    calcium 101
    dairy group 42
    vitamin K 99
bulgur
    food label 26
    grains group 23
bulimia, eating disorders 325
"The Buzz on Energy Drinks" (CDC) 209n

C

caffeine
    blood glucose 304
    eating out 192
    energy drinks 211
    fat burners 217
    foodborne illnesses 322
    overview 209–13
"Caffeine" (The Nemours Foundation/
  KidsHealth®) 209n
caffeine sensitivity 209
calcium
    bone disorders 91
    celiac disease 294
    dairy group 42
    dietary supplements 132
    eating habits 274

calcium, *continued*
    food myths 245
    lactose intolerance 309
    overview 101–6
    percent daily value (%DV) 19
    smart eating tips 340
    tabulated *168*
    veganism 222
    vitamin D 89
    vitamin K 98
    zinc 116
"Calcium" (ODS) 101n
"Calcium and Vitamin D: Important at Every Age"
  (NIAMS) 273n
Calcium Quiz—What's Your Calcium Intake?,
  website address 346
calorie balance, eating pattern limits 6
calories
    added sugars **4**, 149
    alcoholic drinks **303**
    ARFID 327
    beverage choices 64
    chromium 121
    defined 177
    fad diets 242
    gluten-free diet 294
    healthy diet pattern 284
    healthy plate 171
    healthy snacking 205
    milk 42
    nutrition facts label 187
    oil, tabulated *57*
    overview 7–10
    percent daily value 17
    saturated fats 277
    sodium intake 141
    sweets 302
    see also empty calories
cancer
    androstenedione 216
    calcium 105
    celiac disease 290
    childhood obesity 286
    effects of folate 75
    fruit and vegetable consumption 275
    iron 110
    physical activity 263
    selenium 124
    vitamin A 71

cancer, *continued*
    vitamin B6 81
    vitamin C 86
    vitamin D 90
    vitamin E 95
carbohydrates
    caloric balance 7
    nutrition facts label 187
    overview 147–9
    whole grains 25
"Carbohydrates" (OWH) 147n
cardiovascular disease
    calcium 105
    dairy products 43
    E. coli O157:H7 infections 321
    fruits and vegetables 87
    obesity 286
    physical activity 261
    poor quality diet 3
    selenium 124
    sodium 279
carotenoids
    childhood obesity 286
    dairy products 43
    physical activities 261
    selenium 124
    sodium 279
    vitamin C 87
    vitamin D 105
carrageenan, tabulated *167*
cataracts
    vitamin C 87
    vitamin E 95
celiac disease
    folate 74
    overview 289–94
    vitamin K 98
"Celiac Disease" (NIDDK) 289n
Celiac Disease Foundation (CDF), contact 343
Center for Nutrition Policy and Promotion (CNPP),
    contact 343
Center for Science in the Public Interest (CSPI),
    contact 343
Centers for Disease Control and Prevention (CDC)
    contact 350
    publications
        alcohol and health 209n
        childhood obesity 283n
        energy drinks 209n
        good eating habits 273n

Centers for Disease Control and Prevention (CDC)
    publications, *continued*
        nitrate and nitrite 273n
        overweight and obesity 283n
        physical activity 261n
        sodium 139n, 273n
        teen BMI 229n
        water and fluid needs 63n
        water fluoridation 63n
        weight management 7n
"Childhood Obesity Facts" (CDC) 283n
"Children's Bone Health and Calcium"
    (NICHD) 101n
cholesterol levels
    dairy group 43
    food labels 15
    limit saturated and *trans* fat 158
    percent daily value (%DV) 20
    physical activities 263
    protein foods 50
    vegetarian benefits 222
    whole grains 24
"Choose the Foods You Need to Grow" (USDA) 339n
"Choosing a Safe and Successful Weight-Loss
    Program" (NIDDK) 247n
"Choosing Foods for Your Family" (NHLBI) 205n
chromium, overview 119–22
"Chromium" (ODS) 119n
color additives
    food ingredients 161
    tabulated *166*
colorectal cancer
    cruciferous vegetables 277
    folate 75
common cold, zinc 117
common cold myth, vitamin C 88
"Community Water Fluoridation" (CDC) 63n
complex carbohydrates
    described 147
    see also starches
complications
    celiac disease 290
    foodborne illnesses 318
computer use, screen time 267
cookbooks, vegan diet 224
corticosteroids, tabulated *122*
Coumadin (warfarin), vitamin K 97
cruciferous vegetables
    cancer risk 277
    described 275

"Cruciferous Vegetables and Cancer Prevention" (NCI) 273n
"Cut Down on Added Sugars" (ODPHP) 151n

D

d-alpha-tocopherol *see* vitamin E
daily allowance, tabulated *56*
daily reference value, food label 21
dairy products
    calcium 102
    coronary heart disease 277
    foodborne illnesses 315
    high-intensity sweeteners 154
    lactose intolerance 42
    selenium **123**
    vegetarians 224
    vitamin A 69
    vitamin B12 **82**
    zinc **116**
dark green leafy vegetables, folate **74**
DASH diet *see* dietary approaches to stop hypertension
dehydration
    caffeine 210
    foodborne illnesses 319
dehydroepiandrosterone (DHEA), sports supplements 216
depression
    described 76
    eating disorders 329
    health fraud 258
    mental health 264
    obesity **287**
dermatitis herpetiformis (DH), described 291
DH *see* dermatitis herpetiformis
DHA *see* docosahexaenoic acid
DHEA *see* dehydroepiandrosterone
"Diabetes Diet and Eating" (NIDDK) 295n
diabetes
    chronic disease prevention 129
    health fraud 257
    salt sensitive 141
    sports supplements 215
    thiamin 79
    vegan 222
    vitamin D 91
diet
    body mass index 234
    bones 341

diet, *continued*
    calcium 101
    calories 14
    carbohydrates 9
    dietary ingredient 134
    fruits 36
    lactose intolerance 310
    nuts 51
    selenium 124
    sodium 142
    vegetables 30
    vitamin A 69
    whole grains 24
diet myths, weight loss 241
dietary fiber
    carbohydrates 148
    chromium 123
    fruits 36
    grains 23, 242
    packaged food 282
    tabulated *13*
    vegetables 30
dietary folate equivalent (DFE), B vitamins 73
dietary guidelines *see Dietary Guidelines For Americans*
Dietary Guidelines For Americans
    childhood obesity 284
    chromium 122
    health facts **144**
    overview 3–6
    sodium 139
"*Dietary Guidelines for Americans 2015–2020 Eighth Edition*—Executive Summary" (ODPHP) 3n
dietary reference intakes (DRI), chromium 120
"Dietary Sources of Energy, Solid Fats, and Added Sugars among Children and Adolescents in the United States" (NCI) 59n
dietary supplement
    age-related macular degeneration 87
    beta-carotene 69
    calcium 104
    folic acid 73
    health fraud 258
    interaction with chromium 122
    magnesium 112
    overview 132–6
    riboflavin 77
    vitamin B6 80
    vitamin K 98
    see also multivitamin/mineral supplements

"Dietary Supplements: What You Need to Know" (FDA) 131n
dietary trade-offs, described 18
dieting
    anorexia 325
    body mass index 234
    high blood pressure 105
    vegans 223
    weight loss 178, 262
Disabled Sports USA (DS/USA), contact 351
discretionary calorie allowance, empty calories 59
disease prevention, overview 273–9
dough strengtheners, tabulated 168
dual energy X-ray absorptiometry (DXA), body mass index 229
%DV see percent daily value
DXA see dual energy X-ray absorptiometry

E

"Eat for a Healthy Heart" (FDA) 281n
Eat Local: Search for Local Produce or Farmers Markets, website address 346
"Eat Smart and Be Active as You Grow" (USDA) 341n
Eating Disorder Referral and Information Center, contact 344
eating disorders
    body image 240
    body mass index 235
    overview 325–31
"Eating Disorders" (The Nemours Foundation/ KidsHealth®) 325n
eating patterns
    binge eating disorder 326
    dietary guidelines 3
    myths 246
"Eating Well While Eating Out" (The Nemours Foundation/KidsHealth®) 191n
electrolytes
    dehydration 319
    foodborne illness 322
empty calories
    overview 59–61
    see also added sugar
emulsifiers
    color ingredients 162
    tabulated 167

energy balance
    childhood obesity 283
    defined 177
    physical activity levels 8
energy drink
    added sugars 151
    overview 209–13
enriched grains, grain group 23
enzyme preparations
    dairy group 42
    tabulated 168
EPA see eicosapentaenoic acid
ephedra, sports supplements 216
epinephrine, food allergy 305
ergogenic aids see sports supplements
Eunice Kennedy Shriver National Institute of Child Health and Human Development (NICHD)
    contact 344
    publication
        children's bone health 101n
exercise-induced food allergy, described 306
eye disorders, vitamin E 95

F

fad diets
    weight loss myths 241
    weight management 235
Farmers Market Search, website address 347
fast food
    childhood obesity 284
    eating out 178
    weight loss myths 243
"Fast-Food Alternatives" (VA) 195n
fat burners, described 217
fat replacers, tabulated 167
fats
    dairy groups 43
    diabetes 302
    nutrients 50
    oils 56
    overview 157–60
FDA see U.S. Food and Drug Administration
fiber
    cancer 276
    carbohydrates 147
    cutting calories 9
    fruits 37

fiber, *continued*
    grains 23
    multivitamin/mineral supplements 129
    nutrients 14
    vegetables 31
    vegetarian diet 222
firming agents, tabulated *168*
flavor enhancers, tabulated *166*
flavors, certified colors 164
flaxseed, omega 3 fatty acids 223
fluids for consumption
    dehydration **320**
    kidney stones 106
fluoridated water, health benefits 64
folate
    cruciferous vegetables 276
    overview 73–83
    tabulated *167*
    vegan 222
"Folate" (ODS) 73n
folic acid
    fruits 36
    grains group 23
    multivitamin/mineral supplements 128
    neural tube defects 75
    vegetables 30
    see also folate
food additive, described 162
food allergy, weight loss programs 249
"Food Allergy: An Overview" (NIAID) 305n
Food Allergy and Research Education, Inc. (FARE), contact 344
Food and Drug Administration (FDA) *see* U.S. Food and Drug Administration
Food and Nutrition Information Center (FNIC), contact 344
food colors, additives 162
food groups, nutrition guide 174
food labels
    added sugars 152
    nondairy sources 103
    overview 11–21
food myths, described 245
food portions, energy 178
food pyramid, depicted *298*
Food Safety and Inspection Service (FSIS), contact 344
food shopping, overview 187–9

"Food Shopping Tips" (NHLBI) 187n
foodborne illness
    additives 162
    overview 315–24
"Foodborne Illnesses" (NIDDK) 315n
fortified breakfast cereals
    calcium 224
    iron 342
    magnesium **112**
    vitamin A **70**
    zinc **116**
fortified food
    calcium 223
    iron **108**
    MVM dietary supplements 129
    pregnant women 25
    thiamin **78**
free radicals
    selenium 123
    vitamin C 85
    vitamin E 93
fruits
    additives 162
    carbohydrates 147
    chromium 120
    dietary guidelines' key recommendations 5
    fast food alternative 195
    food pyramid **298**
    foodborne illness 318
    health benefits 31
    healthy eating 174, 300
    healthy meal, tabulated *184*
    lower blood pressure 106
    osteoporosis prevention 275
    overview 35–9
    vegan diet 224
    vitamin A **70**
    vitamin C **86**
    vitamin K **97**
"Fruit and Vegetable Consumption" (NCI) 273n
Fruits and Veggies Matter Interactive Tools, website address 347

G

gases, tabulated *168*
gelatin
    animal byproducts 221

gelatin, *continued*
    dietary supplement label 134
    tabulated *166*
generally recognized as safe (GRAS), food
  additive 163
genes
    body shape 235
    weight factor 243
Get Moving! Calculate the Number of Calories
  Burned, website address 346
Girls Health, contact 351
Girl's Health: Nutrition, website address 346
glucose tolerance factor, chromium 119
gluten, celiac disease 289
gluten-free, celiac disease treatment 290
grains
    celiac disease 293
    dietary guidelines' key recommendations 5
    facts 242
    fiber 148
    folate 74
    good nutrition 255
    healthy eating style 174
    healthy heart 281
    healthy lunch guideline 202
    magnesium 112
    overview 23–7
    vegans 224
GRAS *see* generally recognized as safe

H

health fraud
    awareness
        overview 257–9
healthy body weight
    avoidant/restrictive food intake disorder 326
    dietary guidelines **4**
healthy cooking tips, described 336
healthy diet
    celiac disease treatment 290
    facts 242
    food labels 11
    fruits 36
    healthy heart 281
    whole grains 25
"Healthy Cooking and Snacking" (NHLBI) 335n
Healthy Dining Finder, website address 347
"Healthy Eating for Vegetarians" (USDA) 221n

healthy eating pattern
    dietary guidelines 3
    sodium intake 139
healthy lunch tips
    checklist 185
    school cafeteria 201
"Healthy Weight" (CDC) 7n
heart disease
    binge eating disorder 330
    calcium 105
    diabetes 295
    eating style 174
    fat 14
    fiber rich diet 37
    folic acid 76
    food choices 281
    high LDL cholesterol 50
    high sodium intake 139
    magnesium 112
    obesity **287**
    physical activity plan 262
    prohormones 216
    reduced-calorie diet 242
    saturated fat 157, 277
    selenium 124
    sweets 302
    vegetarian diets 222
    vitamin E 95
    whole grains 25
"Heart-healthy Eating" (NHLBI) 273n
heme iron
    anemia 25, 51
    intake 107
    sources **108**
hemochromatosis, defined 88
hemoglobin, iron 107
hemolytic uremic syndrome (HUS), described 320
herbs
    dietary supplements 131
    food flavor 161, 302
    sports supplements 215
heredity, body shape 235
hGH *see* human growth hormone
high blood pressure *see* hypertension
high-fructose corn syrup
    added sugars 149, 188
    food label 27
high-intensity sweeteners, overview 153–5
"High-Intensity Sweeteners" (FDA) 153n

homocysteine, folic acid 76
honey
    blood glucose 297
    food label 27, 152
    vegan 222
"How to Spot Health Fraud" (FDA) 257n
"How to Understand and Use the Nutrition Facts
    Label" (FDA) 11n
human growth hormone (hGH), athletes 216
humectants, tabulated *168*
HUS *see* hemolytic uremic syndrome
hydrogen breath test, described 309
hypertension
    calcium 106
    sodium 144, 278
    vitamin D 91

I

IDEA Health & Fitness Association, contact 351
immune system
    celiac disease 289
    foodborne illness 318
    milk allergy 308
    vitamin A 69
    vitamin C 85
    whole grains 25
    zinc 115, 223
"Improving Your Eating Habits" (CDC) 273n
Institute of Food Technologists, contact 344
insulin
    chromium 119
    defined 295
    magnesium 112
    obesity **287**
International Fitness Association (IFA),
    contact 351
International Food Information Council (IFIC)
    Foundation, contact 344
International Health, Racquet & Sportsclub
    Association (IHRSA), contact 351
iron
    defined 51
    gluten-free diet 294
    MVM supplements 128
    nutrition facts labels 342
    overview 107–10
    refined grains 23
    sources, tabulated *246*

iron, *continued*
    vegetarian food sources 223
    vitamin C 85
"Iron" (ODS) 107n
iron-deficiency anemia, heme iron 25, 51

K

Kidnetic, website address 347
kidney disease, salt sensitive people 141
kidney stones
    calcium oxalate 106
    potassium 31
Kids.gov, website address 351
KidsHealth®, website address 351

L

"Labeling and Nutrition" (FDA) 139n
lactase enzyme, defined 311
lactose-free alternative, lactose intolerance 45
lactose intolerance
    calcium culprits 274
    gluten-free diet 292
    overview 307–13
"Lactose Intolerance" (NIDDK) 307n
LDL *see* low-density lipoprotein
leavening agents, defined 162
"Let's Eat for the Health of It" (USDA) 171n
loperamide (Imodium) 322
low blood glucose, physical activity plan 297
low-density lipoprotein (LDL) cholesterol, defined 50
low-fat milk
    dairy group 42
    healthy choices, tabulated *199*
    riboflavin sources 77
    strong bones 179, 341
    weight loss 242
lutein 276

M

magnesium
    grains 24
    overview 111–3
    vegetarian diets 222
"Magnesium" (ODS) 111n

"Make Better Beverage Choices" (USDA) 63n
maltose, added sugars 27, 149
meal plans
    diabetes 298
    skipping meals 181
    weight-loss program 249
meal myths, described 242
meals
    calcium supplements 105
    dairy products 44
    dietary supplements 131
    guidelines 281
    low-calorie options 244
    processed foods 180
    school cafeteria 201
    sodium intake 141
    vegan diets 224
    whole grains 25
medications
    caffeine 209
    depression 76
    foodborne illness treatment 322
    gluten source 292
    interaction with chromium 122
    interaction with magnesium 113
    interaction with vitamin K 99
    osteoporosis program 275
    performance enhancers 215
megaloblastic anemia, folate deficiency 75
mental health
    benefits of physical activity 261
    eating disorders 329
    self-esteem 237
metabolic syndrome
    benefits of physical activity 261
    obesity **287**
migraine
    low magnesium levels 113
    prevention, riboflavin supplements 78
    treatment, caffeine 210
milk
    calcium source 223
    daily calcium 102
    dairy group 41
    fats 158
    healthy eating pattern 5
    healthy meal 184
    nutrients 65
    saturated fat 158

milk, *continued*
    strong bones 179
    vitamin D sources **90**
    weight loss 242
    see also lactose intolerance
minerals
    grains 24
    overview 119–25
    see also multivitamin/mineral (MVM)
    supplements
monosodium glutamate (MSG)
    food additive 143
    tabulated *166*
monounsaturated fats, product labels 282
MSG *see* monosodium glutamate
multivitamin/mineral supplements,
    overview 127–30
"Multivitamin/Mineral Supplements" (ODS) 127n
MVM *see* multivitamin/mineral supplements
myoglobin, iron 107
MyPlate
    described 173
    food groups 342
    website address 347
"MyPlate" (USDA) 171n

N

National Academy of Sports Medicine (NASM),
    contact 351
National Alliance for Youth Sports (NAYS), contact
    351
National Association for Health and Fitness
    (NAHF), contact 351
National Association of Anorexia Nervosa and
    Associated Disorders (ANAD), contact 345
National Cancer Institute (NCI)
    publications
        cruciferous vegetables and cancer 273n
        dietary sources of energy 59n
        fruits and vegetables 273n
National Center for Complementary and Alternative
    Medicine (NCCAM), contact 345
National Coalition for Promoting Physical Activity
    (NCPPA), contact 352
National Diabetes Education Program (NDEP),
    contact 345
National Eating Disorders Association (NEDA),
    contact 345

National Heart, Lung, and Blood Institute (NHLBI)
    contact 345
    publications
        fast-food alternatives 195n
        food shopping 187n
        healthy cooking 335n
        healthy eating for heart 273n
        healthy snacks 205n
        screen time reduction 267n
National Institute for Fitness and Sport (NIFS), contact 352
National Institute of Allergy and Infectious Diseases (NIAID)
    publication
        food allergy 305n
National Institute of Arthritis and Musculoskeletal and Skin Diseases (NIAMS)
    publication
        calcium and vitamin D 273n
National Institute of Diabetes and Digestive and Kidney Diseases (NIDDK)
    publications
        celiac disease 289n
        diabetes 295n
        foodborne illnesses 315n
        healthy eating 177n
        lactose intolerance 307n
        smart snacks 205n
        weight-loss and nutrition myths 241n
        weight-loss program 247n
National Institutes of Health (NIH), contact 352
National Recreation and Park Association (NRPA), contact 352
National Strength and Conditioning Association (NSCA), contact 352
The Nemours Foundation/KidsHealth®
    publications
        body image and self-esteem 237n
        caffeine 209n
        eating disorders 325n
        eating out 191n
        right weight 233n
        school lunch 201n
        screen time 267n
        sports supplements 215n
        vegan food 221n
        weight gain 253n
neotame
    high-intensity sweeteners 154
    tabulated *165*

neural tube defects
    described 75
    grain 25
    nutrients 31
niacin
    B vitamins 24
    MVM dietary supplements 128
    tabulated *167*
NIDDK *see* National Institute of Diabetes and Digestive and Kidney Diseases
nitrates, described 279
non-dairy calcium choice, milk products 45
non-heme iron, health benefits 51
non-starchy vegetables 195
nutrient claims, described 144
nutrient density, guidelines **4**
"Nutrients And Health Benefits" (USDA) 157n
nutrition
    calcium 274
    described 222
    fruits and vegetables 202
    lactose intolerance 310
    MyPlate 173
Nutrition Explorations, website address 347
nutrition facts label
    food label 53
    iron 342
    nutritional value 32
    overview 11–21
    sodium 139
Nutrition.gov, website address 347
nutritional value
    color ingredients 162
    fruits 37
nuts and seeds, protein foods group 48

O

obesity
    body mass index 230
    healthy eating style 174
    nutrients 24
Obesity Society, contact 345
Office of Dietary Supplements (ODS)
    contact 345
    publications
        calcium 101n
        chromium 119n
        folate 73n

Office of Dietary Supplements (ODS)
    publications, *continued*
        iron 107n
        magnesium 111n
        multivitamin/mineral supplements 127n
        riboflavin 73n
        selenium 119n
        thiamin 73n
        vitamin A 69n
        vitamin B6 73n
        vitamin B12 73n
        vitamin C 85n
        vitamin D 89n
        vitamin E 93n
        vitamin K 97n
        zinc 115n
Office of Disease Prevention and Health Promotion (ODPHP)
    publications
        added sugars 151n
        dietary guidelines 2015–2020 summary 3n
Office on Women's Health (OWH)
    publication
        carbohydrates 147n
oils
    healthy eating pattern 5
    overview 55–7
    tabulated *165*
    vitamin E **94**
omega-3 fatty acids
    described 223
    seafood 50
    see also alpha linolenic acid; docosahexaenoic acid; eicosapentaenoic acid
osteoporosis
    caffeine 210
    calcium 105
    celiac disease 290
    described 98
    vitamin D 89
ounce-equivalent, protein foods group 48
over-the-counter (OTC)
    calcium dietary supplements 104
    foodborne illnesses 322
    sports supplements 215
    zinc dietary supplements 116
"Overview of Food Ingredients, Additives, and Colors" (FDA) 161n

overweight
    body mass index 234
    bulimia 326
    calories 14
    childhood obesity 283
    healthy eating style 174
    tabulated *230*
"Overweight and Obesity" (CDC) 283n

P

pancreas
    childhood obesity 286
    creatine 216
    fruit and vegetable 275
parasite
    described 317
    foodborne illnesses 322
peas
    complex carbohydrates 147
    folate **74**
    healthy eating pattern 5
    iron **108**
    starchy vegetables 196
    tabulated *50*
    vegetables 33
PE Central, contact 352
percent daily value (%DV)
    described 17
    nutrition facts label 187
pernicious anemia, vitamin B12 82
Personal Nutrition Planner from Meals Matter, website address 347
pH control agents, tabulated *168*
phenylalanine, high-intensity sweeteners 154
phenylketonuria (PKU), high-intensity sweeteners 154
phosphate
    calcium dietary supplements 104
    tabulated *168*
physical activity
    blood glucose levels 296
    caloric balance 8
    healthy eating style 174
    healthy habits 255
    osteoporosis 105
    overview 261–5
    overweight 235

physical activity, *continued*
 protein foods group 47
 strong bones 341
 weight-loss program 248
"Physical Activity and Health" (CDC) 261n
Physical Activity Guidelines for Americans ,
 behavior 284
"Pinching Pennies" (NHLBI) 195n
PKU *see* phenylketonuria
PMS *see* premenstrual syndrome
polyunsaturated fats, oils 55
portion size
 cutting calories 9
 food myths 245
 smart snacks 205
potassium
 dehydration 319
 nutrition 222
 nutritional value 37
 restaurant food 282
 vegetables 30
pregnancy
 chromium levels 121
 iron 109
 neural tube defects 75
 nutrition 222
prehypertension, health facts 144
premenstrual syndrome (PMS), described 81
preservatives
 ingredients 134
 tabulated *165*
President's Council on Fitness, Sports, and Nutrition
 (PCFSN), contact 352
protein
 calcium culprits 274
 caloric balance equation 7
 celiac disease 289
 described 223
 high-energy foods 179
 magnesium 111
 nutrition facts label 187
 tabulated *166*
 vitamin B12 82
protein foods group, overview 47–54
puberty
 eating disorders 329
 healthy habits 255
 overweight 235
pyridoxine, vitamin B6 dietary supplements 80

Q

"Questions and Answers on Dietary Supplements"
 (FDA) 131n
quinoa, celiac disease 293

R

RAE *see* retinol activity equivalents
Rate Your Restaurant Diet, website address 347
RDA *see* recommended dietary allowance
RDI *see* recommended daily intake
recipes
 cooking tips 336
 heart healthy 281
 saturated fat 159
 whole grains 26
recommended dietary allowance (RDA)
 chromium 120
 multivitamin and mineral supplements 127
recommended daily intake (RDI)
 calories 13
 chromium 120
 high blood pressure 105
 vitamin A 69
 vitamin D 90
red blood cells
 grains 25
 hemolytic uremic syndrome 320
 iron 107
 vegan 223
 vegetables 31
"Reduce Screen Time" (NHLBI) 267n
refined grains
 carbohydrates 148
 grains group 23
 myths 242
 school cafeteria 202
refractory celiac disease, defined **290**
regulations
 additives 164
 community environment 284
 dietary supplements 134
 sports supplements 215
rennet
 tabulated *168*
 vegetarians 222
retinol, vitamin A 69

retinol activity equivalents (RAE), vitamin A 69
retinyl acetate *see* preformed vitamin A
retinyl palmitate *see* preformed vitamin A
riboflavin
    described 77
    grains group 23
    tabulated *167*
    vegan 222
"Riboflavin" (ODS) 73n
rickets, vitamin D 89
Rolaids®, calcium dietary supplements 104

S

saccharin
    sweeteners
        tabulated *165*
salt sensitive, described 141
saturated fat
    described 157
    dietary guidelines **4**
    food label 53
    healthy eating style 174
    heart-healthy eating 277
    lean proteins 49
    losing weight 242
    low-fat dairy food 43
    oils 55
    packaged food label 282
    sauces/seasonings 32
    solid fats 172
    vegetarian diets benefits 222
"Saturated, Unsaturated, and *Trans* Fats" (USDA) 157n
school cafeteria
    eating, overview 201–3
    healthy choices 191
"School Lunches" (The Nemours Foundation/ KidsHealth®) 201n
screen time, overview 267–9
seafood
    daily recommended intake, tabulated *49*
    eating out 192
    food choices 52
    foodborne illnesses 316, 320
    healthy eating pattern 5
    heart-healthy eating 281
    iron **108**
    MyPlate recommendation 171

seafood, *continued*
    protein group 47
    reducing sodium consumption 145
    selenium **123**
    zinc **116**
seasonings
    fat/calories/cholesterol 32
    sodium consumption 145
selenium
    described 123
    whole grains 25
"Selenium" (ODS) 119n
serving size
    beverage 65
    described 11
    food shopping 187
    healthy teen snack 206
"Should I Gain Weight?" (The Nemours Foundation/ KidsHealth®) 253n
simple carbohydrate, described 147
simple sugars *see* simple carbohydrates
"6 Tip-offs to Rip-offs: Don't Fall for Health Fraud Scams" (FDA) 257n
SmallStep, contact 352
"Smart Shopping for Veggies and Fruits" (USDA) 187n
snacks
    fruits 38
    healthy family snacks 335
    lactose 312
    nuts 225
    sodium 140, 145
    whole grains 26
Society of Health and Physical Educators (SHAPE America), contact 353
sodas
    added sugar calories 149
    eating smart 339, 341
    healthy lifestyle tips 185
sodium bicarbonate, food ingredient 143
sodium chloride, described 139
sodium-free, tabulated *144*
sodium intake
    blood pressure 144
    dietary guidelines **4**
    food selection tips 48
    importance of reducing 139
    nuts 51
    processed and restaurant food 279
    processed meats 53
    sources 140

sodium nitrite
    food ingredient 143
    preservatives, tabulated *165*
"Sodium: The Facts" (CDC) 273n
"Sodium: Q and A" (CDC) 139n
solid fats
    described 56, 180
    examples, tabulated *172*
    plant oils 55
    reducing 172
Spark Teens, website address 347
SPF *see* sun protection factor
spices
    chromium sources **120**
    food additives for taste 162
    sodium alternative 145, 172
    tabulated *166*
sports supplements
    overview 215–9
    see also dietary supplements
"Sports Supplements" (The Nemours Foundation/
    KidsHealth®) 215n
stabilizers
    food additives for texture 162
    gluten-containing additive
    tabulated *167*
starches
    complex carbohydrates 147
    described 298
starchy vegetables
    healthy choices 196
    tabulated *30*
    vegetable subgroup 29
    vitamin B6 source **80**
statistics
    alcoholic beverages 212
    child calcium consumption 102
    child obesity 283
    CVD risk factors in obese children **287**
    E. coli O157:H7 and HUS 320
    eating disorders 325
    energy drinks in schools **213**
    hypertension in children **144**
    physical activity and mortality 265
    screen time 267
    sugar-sweetened beverage 285
"Step 1: Learn about Diabetes" (NIDDK) 295n
stool acidity test 309

sucralose
    FDA-approved sweeteners 154
    sweeteners, tabulated *165*
sucrose
    added sugars 21, 149, 188
    sweeteners, tabulated *165*
sugars
    beverages 64, 211
    calories 7
    carbohydrates 147
    chromium **120**
    dietary guidelines **4**
    empty calories 59
    magnesium 112
    milk products 42
    nutrients without %DV 20
    nutrition facts label 187
    packaged fruits 37
    processed foods 282
    weight loss 242
    see also added sugars
sun protection factor (SPF) 90
sunlight
    extreme sensitivity 81
    vitamin D 90, 223, **311**
supplements
    avoidant/restrictive food intake disorder 327
    caffeine interaction 210
    folic acid 25, 36, 75
    riboflavin 77
    risks 130
    thiamin 79
    vitamin C for cold **88**
    see also dietary supplements; multivitamin/
    mineral supplements; sports supplements
sweeteners
    food additives for taste 162
    tabulated *165*
symptoms
    food allergy 306
    foodborne illnesses 318
    iron deficiency 109
    lactose intolerance 308

T

table sugar *see* sucrose
"Take Charge of Your Health: A Guide for Teens"
    (NIDDK) 177n

"Technology: 5 Ways To Reboot Yourself" (The Nemours Foundation/KidsHealth®) 267n
television usage
    eating at home 179
    health frauds 257
    screen time 182, 267
    weight-loss advertising 247
"Ten Smart Snacks for Teens" (NIDDK) 205n
tests
    A1C 296
    foodborne illness 322
    ketone 304
    lactose intolerance 309
texturizers, tabulated *167*
therapy
    anemia 109
    eating disorder 331
thermogenics *see* fat burners
thiamin
    described 78
    refined grains 23
"Thiamin" (ODS) 73n
thickeners
    food additives for texture 162
    tabulated *167*
thyroid disease, selenium 125
"Toxic Substances Portal-Nitrate and Nitrite" (CDC) 273n
trans fat
    described 158
    food sources 278
    healthy eating pattern 5
    nutrients without %DV 20
    solid fats 180
Tums®, over-the-counter antacid 104

U

upper daily limits 16
USDA *see* U.S. Department of Agriculture
U.S. Department of Agriculture (USDA)
    contact 345
    publications
        added sugars 151n
        beverage choices 63n
        dairy group 41n
        eat smart and be active 341n
        foods for growth 339n
        fruit group 35n

U.S. Department of Agriculture (USDA)
    publications, *continued*
        grains group 23n
        healthy eating 171n, 221n
        MyPlate nutrition guide 171n
        nutrient benefits 157n
        oils 55n
        protein foods group 47n
        saturated and unsaturated fats 157n
        vegetable group 29n
        veggies and fruits shopping 187n
U.S. Department of Veterans Affairs (VA)
    publication
        fast-food alternative 195n
U.S. Food and Drug Administration (FDA)
    contact 345
    publications
        dietary supplements 131n
        food ingredients and additives 161n
        health fraud 257n
        heart-healthy eating 281n
        high-intensity sweeteners 153n
        labeling and nutrition 139n
        nutrition facts label 11n

V

vegan
    described 221
    healthy eating, overview 221–5
"Vegan Food Guide" (The Nemours Foundation/ KidsHealth®) 221n
vegetables
    cruciferous 275
    healthy eating pattern 5
    healthy ways of eating 300
    lunch tips 202
    overview 29–33
Vegetarian Resource Group (VRG), contact 346
vegetarians
    healthy eating, overview 221–5
    protein choices 52
    weight loss myth 245
virus
    described 317
    vitamin D 89
vitamin A, overview 69–72
"Vitamin A" (ODS) 69n

vitamin A deficiency
    common symptoms **71**
    xerophthalmia 79
vitamin B
    blood homocysteine 80
    chromium level enhancer 121
    overview 73–83
    refined grain 23, 242
vitamin B6, overview 79–81
"Vitamin B6" (ODS) 73n
vitamin B12, overview 82–3
"Vitamin B12 Fact Sheet for Consumers" (ODS) 73n
vitamin C
    chemotherapy interaction 87
    fruits and vegetables 179
    iron 108
    overview 85–8
    simple carbohydrates 147
"Vitamin C" (ODS) 85n
vitamin D, overview 89–91
vitamin D deficiency 223
"Vitamin D Fact Sheet for Consumers" (ODS) 89n
vitamin E
    chemotherapy interaction 95
    oils 159
    overview 93–6
"Vitamin E Fact Sheet for Consumers" (ODS) 93n
vitamin K, overview 97–9
"Vitamin K" (ODS) 97n

W

warfarin, vitamin K 99
water
    eating out 192
    eating smart 339
    overview 63–6
    sodium 144
"Water and Nutrition" (CDC) 63n
Weight-Control Information Network (WIN),
    contact 346
weight gain
    anorexia 325
    behavior 284
    creatine 217
weight loss
    cutting calories 9
    diet 178
    eating habits 273
    gluten-free diet 293

weight loss, *continued*
    overview 241–6
    vitamin D 91
"Weight-Loss and Nutrition Myths" (NIDDK) 241n
weight management
    caloric balance 7
    dietitian 235
    water 64
    whole grains 25
"What Are Added Sugars?" (USDA) 151n
"What's the Right Weight for My Height?" (The
    Nemours Foundation/KidsHealth®) 233n
whey
    lactose 313
    tabulated *167*
whole grains
    carbohydrates 148
    folate **74**
    healthy choices 196
    healthy eating pattern 5
    high-energy foods 179
    magnesium **112**
    restaurant food 282
    thiamin **78**
    zinc **116**
Womenshealth.gov, contact 353
Women's Sports Foundation (WSF), contact 353

X

xerophthalmia, vitamin A 71

Y

yeast nutrients, tabulated *168*

Z

zeaxanthin, cruciferous vegetables 276
zinc
    age-related macular degeneration 87
    calcium 106
    described 223
    eye disorders 95
    food myths 245
    immune system 51
    interaction with calcium 106
    overview 115–8
"Zinc" (ODS) 115n